ACHIEVING THE QUADRUPLE AIM OF HEALTHCARE

Agency from the Trenches

Donald E Paxton, MD

We encourage your input; please share your thoughts, ideas, criticisms, etc., through Dr. Paxton's website: DonPaxtonMD.com

About the Author

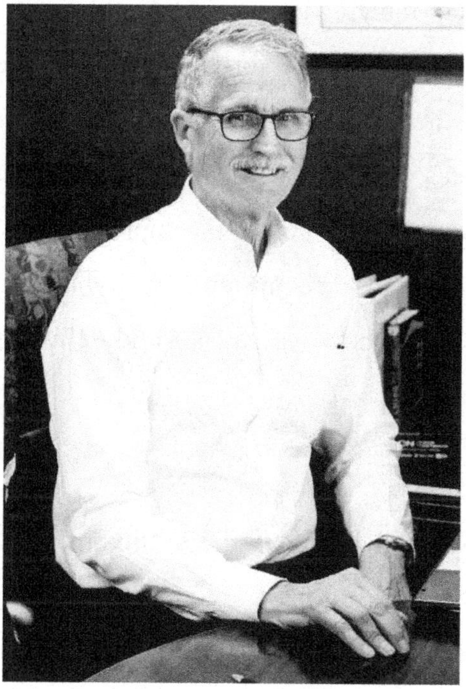

Don Paxton, a Princeton alum, graduated from the University Of Arizona College Of Medicine in 1976. He has practiced general internal medicine in Phoenix for forty-four years. He is married and has three adult daughters.

Endorsements

"Dr. Paxton expertly diagnoses the problems of our corporate health care system which works to enrich Wall Street, rather than save lives. I agree with his prescription to eliminate for-profit insurance companies and adopt the quadruple aim for all health care in the United States. This is an important book in the ongoing conversation about how to improve our woefully inadequate health care system, from how we educate future doctors to how we pay for and deliver health care to Americans."

-Mr. Wendell Potter

Mr. Wendell Potter is the author of *DEADLY SPIN,* a critique of our health insurance companies, and the leader of Center for Health and Democracy, an organized force to examine our healthcare system.

This is a wise summary of what's ailing healthcare from a primary care physician who has lived through the changes and knows we can do better. Don Paxton captures the biggest challenges facing physicians and recommends remedies everyone can use to encourage change. This book is an accessible must-read as all of us will be patients one day.

- Dr Wendy Dean

Dr Wendy Dean is the author of *IF I BETRAY THESE WORDS*, and the founder of the non-profit organization, Moral Injury in Healthcare, which argues that much of what is wrong with healthcare stems from providers being forced to make decisions at odds with their moral compass.

Acknowledgements

Many people assisted me in the development of this book, and I thank them — particularly my editor, Ms. Terry Ratner. The input, support and patience from my wife, Karen, has been invaluable. The ready and "been there" advice from Dr. John Shufelt guided my way. I especially want to thank Sister Margaret McBride and Dr. Charles Daschbach, who have encouraged me for years. Ms. Rhonda Paschal and David Tierney J.D. were "ruthless" proofreaders, teaching me a lot in the process.

Dedication

This book is dedicated to Tinsley Harrison, MD, a seventh-generation physician, who was a major contributor to the advances in medicine in the 20th century. He was the editor of the first five editions of Harrison's Principles of Internal Medicine, the bible of internists everywhere. In the preface to the first edition in 1950, he wrote these profound words.

"No greater opportunity or obligation can fall to the lot of a human being than to be a physician. In the care of the suffering he needs technical skill, scientific knowledge, and human understanding. He who uses these with courage, humility, and wisdom will provide a unique service for his fellow man and will build an enduring edifice of character within himself. The physician should ask of his destiny no more than this, and he should be content with no less."

This book is also dedicated to Dr. Howard Kimball, a general surgeon I met upon returning to Arizona, after finishing my residency at the University of Mississippi in 1979. "Kimball" is a common name in the Latter-Day Saint community. Howard was an offshoot of that community; in Arizona he would be called a Jack Mormon. He smoked cigarettes and could cuss with the best of them. He was a confident old-time surgeon and, if pressed, he could argue that a white piece of paper was black. He cared about his patients and the practice of medicine. He drove to the hospital twice daily for rounds and frequently, I saw him standing at the bedside, cutting up the meat for his post-op patients and encouraging them. He taught me a lot about treating and managing patients in the nonacademic world of medicine.

Once he caught me in a meeting with some visiting medical businessmen. After gathering where that meeting was headed, he only shook his head, and walked away in disgust. He was right. It turns out the paper was black.

Table of Contents

Chapter One

Introduction

Is healthcare important? You bet your life it is. You bet your life, and the lives of your loved ones, whenever you engage with our healthcare system. As you will see, the American healthcare system is defective in major ways. Many times our experience of medicine is gratifying, but clearly, there are problems. I am interested in healthcare reform and certainly it is time for change. As one of my bright attorney patients succinctly said, “There are problems with healthcare wherever you look. Healthcare is on fire.” Right. She is a bankruptcy attorney.

I write these words on Sunday, November 1st, 2020 two days before that election, Biden vs. Trump. Everyone, both right and left, is anxious to know the outcome and worried that the other side will win. The sun will continue to rise, no matter the winner. Human affairs will continue to lurch forward in surprising ways, and we will manage. The Covid-19 pandemic will gradually be controlled by natural forces, our social forces, and science. Other major problems remain in front of us. The intelligence we bring to our decision making is important. The courage we bring to what we do and say publicly is even more important, and that includes our healthcare system.

This book is about healthcare reform. There are major issues in many aspects of American medicine, such as cost and coverage. I cover these broader areas, but I do not address the clinical management of specific conditions.

Clearly, doctors and medical procedures at times lead to poor outcomes. Much has already been written about improving the hows and whats of the specific care given. These are areas I do not address.

The ideas presented in this book will be controversial at best, some radical. I am a centrist. Both the capitalistic right and the socialistic left may be offended, yet each view brings elements of truth that add to the whole. An open-minded consideration of these ideas may help move our healthcare in the right direction.

Reform is about change. The inertia of the status quo is powerful in medicine as precedent holds a great deal of weight. However, clinging to "how it has always been done" has been a medical disaster at times. An even greater problem is the desire of the financial forces involved in medicine, the "medical industrial complex," to keep things exactly as they are. They have a great deal of influence in our government. A government for the people needs to hear from the people. Have the courage to say and do. The American experiment begs for it.

Acknowledging the truths on both sides of a debate should help calm emotions and invite mindful solutions. The arrogance of Ms. Clinton referring to President Trump's base as "deplorables" is as offensive as the term "losers" Trump used to describe American soldiers. The fact is Trump's administration pursued Covid-19 vaccines with vigor, which benefited our nation, just as the Biden administration's emphasis on promoting the use of those vaccines was advantageous in lowering the number of deaths, and illnesses from Covid. From a centrist view, both actions are to be applauded.

The fact that we all make mistakes is a given. It is a key part of progress. A book by Kathryn Schulz, *Being Wrong,*[1] covers this reassuring point in detail. These errors need clear-minded examination and forgiveness for us to move forward. Absolution and open-mindedness do not have the same juice as clenched jaw positionalism, but issues demanding healthcare reforms are beyond urgent, and need our unbiased attention. Our responses must be creative, educated, carefully thought out, ethical, strong, and mature.

There are so many issues clamoring for resolution. A conceptualization called the quadruple aim has arisen as one way of sorting out these problem areas. It began as the triple aim formulated in 2008, by Dr. Don Berwick [2], with the Institute for Healthcare Improvement (IHI). These initial three aims were to improve the patient experience of healthcare, to address the uncontrolled expense of healthcare, and to provide healthcare for our entire population. A fourth aim, to improve the physician experience and decrease burnout, was added by Drs. Christine Sinsky and Thomas Bodenheimer [3], in 2014. These four goals comprise the quadruple aim.

All four goals may not be in the foreground, when making medical decisions in the exam rooms, but they are present in the background. All four goals should absolutely be present, and discussed when bureaucracies are discussing policy. Financial integrity, patient experience, population health, and provider well-being are all important, and somewhat conflicting goals. These four aims and their conflicts need to be considered in each instance of system decision making because a decision in one area impacts all the areas. For instance, a decision to ignore physician wellbeing certainly undermines the stability needed to achieve population health, the quality of the patient experience, and ultimately the financial wellbeing of the system.

Now a word about me; I love the practice of medicine. I find meaning in sitting with patients, new or old, in a quiet room listening to their story, their problems, and helping them formulate a way forward. One foot must be thoroughly grounded in unblinking science, and the other open to our common humanity. And the delivery must be founded in trust and respect, at times surprisingly frank and honest, and always tempered by human kindness.

My practice is general internal medicine, a nonsurgical field focusing on adults over eighteen years old. I grew up in Scottsdale, Arizona, and went to Medical School at the University of Arizona in Tucson. After graduation in 1976, I moved to Jackson, Mississippi, for my internship, and residency at the University of Mississippi Hospital. Now in my 44th year of practice, I have been located in downtown Phoenix, Arizona since 1979.

In Jackson I met my outstanding wife, Karen, the director of a quite successful Montesorri school in Phoenix. Her first job as a teenager was being a stable hand on a horse ranch, mucking stalls. At age 21, while pregnant with our first child, she was elected foreman of the jury in a murder trial. They found the defendant guilty.

My oldest daughter, Kate, is a nurse practitioner midwife, who attends home births, co-owns a birthing center, and performs artificial insemination. She delivered her first child in my dining room in a Lamaze (water) tub at age forty. She labored kneeling on her hands and knees. When it was time to deliver, rolling over onto her haunches, she reached down in the water, and pulled up her son by herself. (Yes, help was in attendance.)

My second daughter, Elizabeth, is a chaplain and the director of a Clinical Pastoral Education program (a training program for chaplains,) in Alexandria, Virginia. Her residency after receiving a theology degree, was at a Level One Trauma Hospital, in Washington, D.C., which led to work as a hospice chaplain. Her two children were born at home with her sister attending.

I delivered my third daughter, Rebecca, in a birthing center. (I am an internist, and would have no business delivering a child alone. An obstetrician was present.) She, now is a fourth year medical student at the University of Arizona College of Medicine - Phoenix (UACOM - Phoenix). She is currently studying on the east coast on her way to becoming a surgeon. Twice she has organized school trips to Tijuana, Mexico, to deliver medical care to the waiting immigrants there; impoverished, resilient, hardworking people, looking for their chance.

I love the practice of medicine, and I love my family more. They are an undeserved blessing.

I would like to make three points. This book is written from the point of view of a practicing primary care physician. Twelve hours a day during the week, and on weekends, I see patients, answer multiple phone calls, wrestle with electronic medical records, and worry about keeping my business afloat, financially. Daily, I am beyond frustrated by pharmaceutical opaqueness and expense, and by the roadblocks thrown up by the insurance companies, trying to minimize their costs. I have spent time in administrative work, on hospital committees, and in physician organizations, as have most doctors, but I am not a research scientist, academician, administrator, or teacher. My thinking is grounded in my study of healthcare reform, and my day-to-day practice of medicine.

Much of what is written about physicians assumes that our aptitudes, job requirements, and patient relations can be rounded into one experience, and the findings applied to all. They cannot. Radiologists and pathologists never deal with live people but provide the factual base the whole system stands on. Research doctors may never see patients, but they supply the ever-expanding knowledge base needed for the advance of medicine. Administrative physicians have a remote history of seeing patients. Their job is to buffer the dictates of our corporate and governmental overlords with the reality of the trenches. Surgeons and other proceduralists may never see the patient prior to the procedure, and afterward for perhaps one additional visit. The requisite bond was accomplished by the advice of the referring physician, the reputation of the institution, or by the financial contracts of the insurance carrier. Emergency physicians must assess rapidly, frequently under emotional circumstances, and their overall assessment is of primary importance. They rarely have follow-up with the patients. Most medical school graduates, two-thirds, go into these supporting fields, and the minority go into primary care fields. Yet the general advice available is presented as if we all had ongoing personal relationships with the patients, which is far from reality. Again, this book is written from the point of view of primary care medicine, and only some of it applies to other specialties.

Most people practicing primary care medicine are family practitioners. My hat is off to them. They can be responsible for the entire spectrum of human ages, birth to death, including all the maladies that may occur in between. They have extensive training in this and develop astute patient management skills. Pediatricians see patients from birth to around age 18. They must always be on the alert for the unusual in the mix of routine childhood diseases, and they become skilled in dealing with parents. My kind of primary care is general internal medicine. Its training post medical school is usually three years and covers all of the main organ systems. The specialists go on to fellowships after those three years, and spend two years becoming gastroenterologists, pulmonologists, rheumatologists, etc. The great majority of medical school graduates who begin post graduate training in internal medicine become specialists, not primary care physicians.

A second point regards the intended audience of the book. It's aimed at medical students, who will forge our future. Remember where you came from and remember kindness. Your importance and cachet is great: do not be intimidated. You absolutely belong here. You are not an imposter. You may think your fortune is great, but it is not as great as your responsibility both to serve your patients, and to use your fresh wisdom for the improvement of healthcare in America. Our medical students with their intelligence, thirst for knowledge, and drive, should not be satisfied with graduating into the rat-race of the American medical industrial complex. Rather, they need to develop into a force for change.

These words are aimed at our medical educators. Your focus on teaching, research, and publishing, is an important link in the network of medicine but may be somewhat insular. These chapters will present systemic problems of healthcare in the United States. I believe part of your responsibility is to be sure your students develop an awareness of what awaits them and to be sure they honor those social values that brought them into medicine in the first place

It is also written for the multitude of us physicians who scurry around under administrative pressures, while carrying life preserving responsibilities. It is aimed at the administrators of medicine, those who manage our hospitals, physician practices, and other healthcare operations. Your job is to enable healthcare, not constrain it. It is written for our governmental representatives. Please use your power with courage and humility, so the future will be proud of your accomplishments. A sixth audience are the patients we presume to serve. Hopefully you will gain insight into the problems of healthcare and voice your opinions.

A third point regards why I am writing this book. It is because the practice of medicine is my life, second only to my family, so this is an act of personal completion.

The forces that maintain the status quo are strong. Commercial medical corporations have much to lose if needed change is wrought, and these industries are committed to not moving forward. We have a battle in front of us as Medicare will be insolvent over the next few years. (The estimates keep changing. I am hearing from 2024 to 2026.). Confronting this reality will bring about another debate regarding our healthcare system – our elected representatives need to hear from our frustrated and medically bankrupt populace, from physicians in offices actively caring for this population, not just from the coalesced administrations of our commercial insurance and pharmaceutical companies. Our government needs to be resolute in forging and maintaining a new path.

Bernie Sanders promoted single-payor healthcare while running for President in 2019 and 2020. At the time the idea seemed kooky to me, but no longer. As this book will demonstrate, chapter by chapter, the sound way forward is through a single payor system. Many commentators in the Wall Street Journal are committed to the current system, but that system only enriches the major insurance companies, their principals, and the stockholders. It is detrimental to each of the quadruple aims.

This book is about healthcare reform. It details how expensive our system is, and why. It will reveal the dreary experience of our physicians, and why so many are leaving the profession. It exposes the impersonal experience of receiving healthcare that our patients face. Remember going to the movies, in a dark quiet theater and when the evils of HMOs are mentioned, the audience breaks into applause. And perhaps our greatest shame, we examine that roughly ten percent of our people either delay healthcare or do not get medical attention due to cost. (4)

Chapter Two

Silos

Have you ever driven through Farm County and noticed flanks of huge concrete silos, hundreds of feet high, with the capacity to store tons of grain, cottonseed, and silage? They are arranged side by side, each with a valve mechanism underneath, an auger, which delivers their contents into trucks pulling up below.

There are multiple organizations in medicine which keep the wheels of our medical industrial complex turning: pharmaceutical and medical device corporations, drug stores and hospital chains, governmental agencies, and, of course, health insurance companies. These corporations are similar to grain silos. They are hierarchical in structure. At the top, is a Board of Directors, then CEOs (chief executive officers) and other corporate officers, including medical directors whose job is to stay attuned to the changing mandates of the Center for Medicare and Medicaid Services (CMS), other governmental agencies, and private health insurance companies. The medical directors are responsible for delivering messages to practicing physicians. Support for the upper level may come from stockholders of the corporation. Beneath the top layer are cadres of assistants, further levels of the administration – nurses and social workers who provide support, and guidelines to the physicians in caring for patients. The patients "belong" to the medical corporations. As in a silo, the highest pressure is on the bottom layer, the physicians, who are expected to carry out the directives of the higher-ups and attend to their patients

There are two large problems. First, the medical silos are not placed side by side, each delivering goods to one truck at a time. Instead, they are arranged as a funnel, so that any one practice, solo or group, may simultaneously be exposed to the different and changing mandates of multiple silos. In my solo practice on any one day, I may be responsible for Medicare fee for service patients, Medicare Advantage patients, Medicaid (AHCCCS in Arizona) and patients from Aetna, Blue Cross/Blue Shield, United HealthCare, CIGNA, and traditional cash patients. Many of these programs may seek to incentivize me by offering financial awards for meeting certain criteria. But each silo has a different set of benchmarks and is obliged to change metrics annually, in part because CMS changes its expectations each year.

As an example, consider Hemoglobin A1c standards. We largely measure the success of diabetic management by drawing A1C blood levels, which correlates closely with the average blood sugar levels over the previous three months. A good A1c is between 4.9 and 5.5. A bad A1c is greater than

7.9. Some insurance companies want the diabetics' A1c less than 7.0, some less than 7.5, and some less than 9.0 percent. Once the goal is established, the provider must then consider medications. In treatment, there are long-acting insulins which help control blood sugars for an entire 24 hours after an injection. Some insurance companies only cover Lantus and others only cover Levemir. Both are good and effective treatments. Which one is covered by the insurance at play? Look it up on the computer. Surely it only takes a few seconds. But too frequently there have been recent contractual changes and the information is not current, or the computers or the electronic medical record system are faltering.

This welter of ever-changing expectations, mandates, and metrics is confusing, distracting, and time consuming. So, while I sit in the office with my 90-year-old patient who suffers with heart failure, diabetes, and hypertension, who is ready to call it quits, and her 65-year-old daughter who is grappling with these problems and beginning to consider the possibility that her mother is right, I am supposed to find a way forward. I'm committed to do the right thing. Please remember that I have a primary care practice to run and employees to pay. It's important for me to know and meet the metrics of her insurance company and those of all the other patients. If I don't earn those incentives, I either go out of business or join the multitude of managed practices run by private concerns, hospitals, health insurance companies, or governmental systems. These practice possibilities are also corporate silos, which bring another layer of unnecessary, distracting and conflicting forces to bear as I sit with my 90 year old patient and her loving daughter with social concerns. This funneling of ever-changing demands from multiple silos does not make sense.

It is important to take time to effectively manage, the nuances of complex visits like this. Trust is essential. I spend time listening to the patient and her daughter, looking them in the eye, giving clear instructions, and speaking a few hard truths about the situation, all of this with compassion. These are the elements needed to create relationships. Using my time to decipher confusing mandates and changing formularies gets in the way of competence, integrity, consistency, and connection, all part of the building blocks of trust. The silos that create the distraction and confusion may look at the sacrifice of trust as unfortunate as collateral damage to some greater good. But there is no greater good, when every patient-physician interaction creates distrust in the provider and in our medical system. Oh right; there is the financial benefit that accrues to the insurance company upper management and to the stockholders. Is that what we really want in healthcare? Is that what you want your doctor visit to be about?

It is important for me to use my spare time to keep up with changes in medical science, rather than learning the new mandates of the day from the various silos. Lifelong study is a noble obligation and part of the physicianship package, we accept, when we matriculate into medical school. I also deserve to maintain physical and spiritual fitness as well as to spend time with my family. Metrics can have a role in promoting quality and continuing improvement, but only if they are uniform, and stable.

A second problem with the American silo arrangement, is that it is just that; an arrangement meant to benefit the decision makers and the stockholders of healthcare and insurance companies more than the beneficiaries of these companies, the patients. "*Deadly Spin*", [(1)] is an excellent resource book written by Wendell Potter which explains the corporate machinations entrenched to maintain the profitability of the medical industrial complex. Potter first began his career as a journalist which evolved into public relations, first with Humana, and later with CIGNA. He rose into the higher corporate ranks and witnessed how the top officers made million-dollar salaries, and the shareholders enjoyed spectacular earnings. All the while the insured were charged high monthly premiums, while they frequently paid out of pocket for less expensive concerns. If a major health issue occurred and deductibles had to be met, bankruptcy would ensue. It is well known that healthcare debt is the largest cause of bankruptcy in the U.S. [(1)] There is an arrangement in American healthcare insurance. It strictly benefits the insurance companies; not the insured.

"Deadly Spin" details how public relation experts working for health insurance companies perpetrate the myth of superiority of American healthcare. Major insurance companies collude to create front organizations that interact with the media and the government in an attempt to influence opinions. Their main argument is that a national single-payor option would be a step towards communism. They bankroll lobbying efforts by the millions to make sure the voting goes their way. Potter points out that in 2009, the ongoing crisis in healthcare financing led President Obama to call a summit in Washington. Government representatives as well as numerous health insurance executives were in attendance. By promising to control expenses and deliver savings via traditional American competition, major healthcare insurance companies were permitted to remain in business.

But it was business as usual, and their "competition" never delivered savings. The fortunes and very lives of the American people are at stake here. It's high time that America puts people ahead of the interests of duplicitous healthcare corporations.

In the 1990s, multiple consolidations occurred. The resulting concentration of power permitted the cornering of the health insurance market by a few cooperative "competitors." The results were lucrative. (3) In the same year, the total compensation for the ten highest paid CEOs at for-profit healthcare insurance companies ranged between $16.5 million and $389.6 million. (2) In 2021, the top director at CMS is estimated to have made less than $350,000. (3)

Most economically advanced nations, except the United States, have single payor systems. (Norway has multiple administrative outlets, but they're all governed by a single set of guidelines and expectations.) It is important and instructive to learn how we got here. It was not contrived by a cabal of right-wing capitalists. Healthcare in the U.S. evolved from a noble - minded effort with integrity and sound values into a huge complex machine with one overriding ethos: strong financial success.

The history of healthcare in the United States has to do with the federated nature of our country. Constitutionally, the majority of power in healthcare affairs resides with the individual states, not with our federal government. By the time the need for a national plan became obvious, private insurance companies had a strong foothold. Think Blue Cross Blue Shield of (you name the state). The following review is taken from an article, "HealthCare Finance Review" in 2005, by Edward Berkowitz, in the National Library of Medicine. [5]

At the beginning of the 20th century, it became apparent that the loss of wages brought on by a serious illness was catastrophic for families. Early efforts at establishing "sickness insurance" at the beginning of the 20th century in the era of Teddy Roosevelt focused on wage replacement. Lost wages were far more disruptive than medical expenses in the early 1900s. These efforts occurred in the state capitals, rather than Washington D.C. Note that in that era the American Medical Association was opposed to health insurance.

During the period of the New Deal, in the 1930s, medical care was becoming more expensive, and the search shifted from insuring against lost wages, to paying for medical expenses. The Social Securities Act of 1935, provided for financial security after retirement, but not for medical care. At the same time, the concept of medical insurance was becoming widespread in Europe, South America, and Asia. The Great Depression of the

1930s, and World War II, in the 1940s, presented more obstacles to a national health plan. In 1945 and 1947, President Harry Truman supported a national universal health insurance for people of all ages. It did not pass, because private health insurance had become more common, and was thought to be sufficient. Again, private health insurance is governed at the state, not national level, reinforcing the model of local control.

By 1957, it was apparent to Congress that due to the rising costs of medical care, older people were presenting a risk for private insurers and needed their own public health coverage program. President John Kennedy supported a Medicare bill in 1961, which did not pass, but negotiations continued revolving around the role private insurers might play, given that they already had an established presence in the field. Insurance to cover physicians' bills as well as hospital fees became part of a conversation, which also focused on the inclusion of the indigent population. Ultimately, in 1965, as part of the Great Society Program, President Lyndon Johnson signed the Medicare and Medicaid Act. It provided coverage for hospital expenses (Part A) and for physician expenses (Part B) for the elderly (Medicare) and the impoverished (Medicaid.) This act continued the participation of private carriers, covering the 20 % copays of Medicare, and it provided for continued state level supervision of the programs. In the 1980s, to help constrain the rising costs of medical care, Medicare Part C was created, financing Medicare Advantage Programs which incorporated features of managed care. A Children's Health Insurance Program (CHIP) was created in 1997 to provide health insurance, and preventative care to children of families making too much to qualify for Medicaid. In 2006, President George Bush, Jr., signed off on Part D Medicare, which provided an optional prescription drug benefit.

In 2010, the Affordable Care Act (ACA or Obamacare) created the Health Insurance Marketplace (commonly referred to as the "exchange" as in stock exchange. "Marketplace" is the preferred term). The ACA includes increased access to health insurance in both the private and public sectors and emphasizes preventive care. It has expanded health insurance coverage to some 20 million people. President Trump sought to abolish the Affordable Care Act in 2017 and was stopped by the Democrats and one Republican senator, John McCain of Arizona.

The silos of for-profit healthcare corporations are presumed to exist to create competition, which is supposed to lead to better and less expensive care. Nothing could be further from the truth. America ranks first in the world in healthcare expense. In 2020, $11,945 was the medium cost per person, per year. The next highest country being Switzerland at $7,136. So where do we rank in terms of quality? For all that money we should be getting something out of it. Per the Commonwealth Fund we are a distant 11th out of 11 first world countries in terms of healthcare quality. [(7)] Worldwide surveys by The World Health Organization says the best healthcare is in Belgium, other European Nations, and Japan. America comes in 30th out of 191 nations. [(8)]

So, aside from its damage to the patient-physician relationship, the for-profit corporate practice of medicine is not only expensive, but largely ineffective. Under the guise of avoiding socialism, under the pretense of creating capitalistic competition, the medical industrial complex gives us second rate healthcare at extorted prices. It guts the American public like a fish.

Dr. Wendy Dean, psychiatrist, has written a great deal about physician burnout. [9] She believes that the main cause of burnout is moral injury. The constraints and incentives of the modern corporate practice of medicine are damaging to the intrinsic morality of physicianship. In an exchange of e- mails, she recently introduced me to the Friedman Doctrine, which holds that the sole obligation of a corporation is to maximize the financial profits of the shareholder. Milton Friedman won the Nobel Prize for Economics in 1976, for his research on monetary theory and stabilization policy. His popularity in MBA programs stems from his assertion that social and moral obligations ought to be ignored by corporations. Their sole and proper role is to make a profit for shareholders. By granting shareholder status to the upper echelons of corporations, including supervisory boards, executive teams, and physician directors, a powerful incentive is created to make decisions which cross over the ethical boundaries of serving their patients first. All of us in medicine have a professional moral heritage (Hippocrates, "first do no harm", Mayo brothers, "The best interest of the patient is the only interest to be considered…") Using physicians like pawns to game the system and maximize corporate financial profit above all else, is beyond repugnant.

Now it is January, 10th 2021, four days after our day of shuddering, the insurrection at the U.S. capitol. Our constitution, God bless its soul, held. Over the next days, weeks, and months we will see how wise the center can be.

I am not a big fan of for-profit corporate forms of medicine, but I do agree that most of our advances in medicine are due to organized group collaborations found among medical schools, university research centers, private industry, organized medicine, and research, funding from NIH. In 2001, a book was published by the Institute of Medicine: *Crossing the Quality Chasm: A New Health System for the 21st Century.* [10] It was a major report, produced by an integrated, multipurpose effort which led to improvement in hospital performance. A number of safety measures were instituted, including pauses prior to surgical procedures and improved patient handoffs. We would not have been able to mount the Covid-19 vaccination program without the contributions of pharmaceutical giants. There are realms of medicine which require the cooperation of many talents.

Where I differ is when the reach of organized group think presumes to extend itself into the privacy and trust of the patient-doctor relationship. One of the first scientific truths, we are taught in college is that you cannot measure anything without interrupting or affecting the results. Leatherman and Berwick acknowledged this truth in a recent article in *The Journal of the American Medical Association* (JAMA). "Accelerating Global Improvements in Healthcare Quality." [11] "Metrics are essential to encourage change and guide improvement, but when such measures are used punitively or impose an excessive data burden, improvement slows." These metrics, as deployed in this last decade, and applied in multiple differing formats because of our silo-ed medical system, have indeed intruded into the interpersonal relationships in doctors' offices. In mid-December of 2020, JAMA published an issue concentrating on trust in medicine. I found one article particularly germane. "Patient Consumerism, Healing Relationships, and Rebuilding Trust in Healthcare," by Khullar and

Darlen. [(12)] "In some respects, healthcare functions like any other industry… Patients are encouraged to behave like consumers by, for example, price shopping and assuming greater financial responsibility for the care they use. Yet, healthcare is also like no other industry. Patients often access health services in times of personal crisis and vulnerability. Relatively large information asymmetries exist between clinicians and patients. There is a moral obligation to care for patients regardless of their ability to pay. Interpersonal relationships remain central to the delivery of high-quality care."

Throughout current medical literature, without great fanfare, this same theme is repeatedly acknowledged. The privileged position of the final judgment of the patient acting on the advice of a trusted, educated, and compassionate physician ought not to be breached. This is a basic granular truth that cannot be summed, and averaged into anything meaningful to the corporate world.

Are there alternatives to the system of multiple silos that have evolved in the United States? Certainly. We are surrounded by them. All other first world countries have single-payor systems that make healthcare available to everyone, at considerable cost savings, and with improvement in quality, and a decrease in opaqueness and confusion. Senator Bernie Sanders made universal healthcare a central part of his campaign to become the Democratic party's presidential candidate during this last election cycle. Bernie was right. We need to get on board.

Take a moment to digest these numbers. The Peterson- Kaiser Family Foundations Health Systems Tracker regularly scans reputable sources for many quality and expense comparisons from across the developed world. It is readily available on the Internet.

The U.S. ranked nineth out of nine comparable countries in terms of access and quality of healthcare in 2016, falling behind the Netherlands, Australia, Sweden, Japan, Austria, Germany, France, and the United Kingdom. In terms of our management of major diseases, we came in ninth out of nine in preventing death. Our maternal mortality rate, 25.6 per 100,000 live births vastly exceeds the 4.6 mortality rate for the countries listed above. Our C-section rate is 30% and in other countries it is less than 5.0 %. Eight percent of our population is uninsured. In countries with universal healthcare, no one is uninsured. We lead the way in healthcare expenditures. In the U.S. we spend $10,637 per individual per year. Other comparable nations spend $5,527 annually. In 2020 our expense was 19.7% of our GNP, at 4.12 trillion dollars.

Interestingly, we have 2.64 doctors per 1000 population, significantly less than the 3.68/ thousand for the rest of the developed world. Our hospitals have as many nurses as other countries, but about twice the number of administrative staff. We lead the world in healthcare expense, our overall quality is embarrassing, and we are pathetic in our care of the underprivileged.

A recent article in JAMA February, 21st 2021, by Dr. Robert Kocher, [(13)] reviews some of the reasons healthcare in the U.S. is so expensive. There is a great deal of waste; estimates range up to 25 percent. The largest category of wasteful spending is administrative. Much of the blame lies with our duplicative fragmented payor systems. Each major plan supports advertising, sales forces, medical directors, systems for claims adjudication, and major administrative hierarchies. Remember the CEOs of major carriers, who earned multiple million-dollar salaries per year while the head administrator of CMS earned less than

$350,000. Note that in 2020, the first year of our pandemic, health insurance costs increased with companies earning record profits, and their administrators banked gluttonous salaries.

A good deal of fighting continues, concerning the future of healthcare. The major carriers want to continue mining this vein of gold indefinitely. How long will that be? Not too long. Best estimates are that healthcare expense will be greater than 20% of our GNP by 2024. The system, as we know it, is in a slow-motion crash. The unfortunate part of this is people will continue to age, get sick, and need healthcare. And many will go without coverage because of the outrageous costs. Disruption lies ahead. Change will and must happen.

The advantages of a single payor system are many. The problems of excessive mandates and metrics, a major dilemma for physicians, should be simplified. We could enforce transparency in pricing of medications and services. Administrative duplication could be eliminated. The long- awaited goal of the electronic medical record (EMR) interoperability could be achieved, and the ideal of universal coverage accomplished.

Now it is February 28, 2021. The Biden administration is beginning to take hold, and the Covid-19 epidemic is declining in the U.S. We are starting to hear national, along with state level buzz for healthcare reform. Naturally, these stirrings for change begin on the progressive left. The conservative right wants to maintain the status quo. Decision makers at the top of the major financial silos, commercial insurances and big pharmaceutical companies, like things just the way they are. They invest a great deal in influencing our lawmakers to keep the current arrangements, which we know have a number of disadvantages for anyone outside the upper tiers of those silos. This debate is approaching and needs to be addressed in the near future. According to the Congressional Budget Office, the Medicare Hospital Insurance Trust Fund becomes insolvent in 2024. (This estimate is shortened from 2026 because of the expense of the pandemic.) Solving this issue requires an increased cash flow or tightening of the belt somewhere in our current healthcare system.

Another way in which the corporate practice of medicine is a bad influence is when doctors themselves, guided by profit mindset, band together to form coalitions. In some circumstances, this is the only way to push back against the dominant power of commercial payors. This can be reasonable, but at times doctors buy into the corporate think of MBAs, in which financial gain is always the motive. A common example is anesthesiology, where anesthesiologists band together in large groups in hospitals or clinics, and corner the market. They can and do demand much higher rates of pay than many other specialties. These coalitions (cartels, really) and the earnings they require contribute to the excessive growth of medical expenses compared to other services in the economy.

Several groups of physicians are underpaid in our current system, especially those doing cognitive work. Psychiatrists and primary care physicians are in this group. One response of the primary care physicians is to offer concierge medicine. This is a fee-for-service model, again guided by a profit motive, in which their patients pay high annual retainer fees in order to receive attentive care, something that occurred for nominal fees in the 20th century. The patient panels of a successful concierge practice will be in the 400-600 range, which requires seeing six to ten clients a day, compared to a traditional family physician's average of 25 patients a day and a panel of 3000 to 5000.

Concierge practices tend to congregate in the wealthier parts of town, and while they offer a fine service to the patients that sign up, they do not serve the less affluent two-thirds of our populace.

Another problem is called surprise billing. The medical industry has created networks of doctors of many specialties which contract with insurance carriers at negotiated prices. If a complex emergency occurs and the patient must be hospitalized, the situation may demand services of providers not in the contracted network who bill at rates far above what the patient expected from their insurance company.

Carrie Colla, PhD, wrote about this phenomenon in a recent JAMA article. (14) "Surprise billing is a result of, and illustrates, many potentially troubling trends in medicine: rapid vertical and horizontal consolidation on the part of healthcare clinicians and systems, accompanying varied and high prices in commercial insurance markets, and private investment in physician groups (physician staffing companies in particular), emergency transportation companies, and hospitals." Regulations of the Biden administration have attempted to put an end to surprise billing. But the mindset remains.

A single-payor system implies the government would be in control. Does this invite communism? Well, the majority of Americans past the age of 65, are already in a healthcare system controlled by the government, called Medicare. Is Medicare communistic? Our VA system and Indian Health Services also are government regulated; do you think they are leading to communism? I have a friend in the health insurance advising business. He relates that many people verbally distain communistic medicine, but the last thing they would want is to do without their Medicare benefits.

Over the past four to five decades the definition of a successful doctor has changed from consideration of how helpful he or she is to their patients, to consideration of their annual income, financial worth, and the location of their residence. All the business advisors that influence the physician: attorneys, accountants, and investment advisors, and the chat in the doctors' lounge, assert an outsized influence on the values of the practice of medicine. Like the freshwater fish gradually accommodating to salt water, we don't even realize it is happening. The values we carried upon being accepted into medical school fade, and are supplanted by the love of money. The for-profit corporate mindset is a destructive influence on the proper way to practice medicine.

The multiple silos we endure are an integral component of this investment mentality. It tears at the heart of the patient-physician relationship, and ignores issues of population health, patient experience, financial soundness, and physician well-being. We medical providers have an obligation to our country to cultivate our original values and call out this influence while our government needs to be bold in constraining it. We need to move toward a single payor healthcare system.

A radical change is in order.

Chapter Three

Agency

Today is April 30th, 2021. It is ten days after Derek Chauvin was found guilty in the death of George Floyd. This homicide occurred on May 25th, 2020, which led to massive protests against police brutality in the treatment of people of color. The protests were unrelenting, and all of these events seemed to have been a watershed moment in our nation's history. The primal sin of our nation seems to be recognized. A huge gash in humanity is admitted. We in medicine need to do our share to help the healing.

Dr. Glen Fogerty has a Ph.D., in education and specializes in the admission process into institutions of higher learning. He has served as the director of admissions into MBA programs, and generally, he found those candidates to be bright, driven to be in charge, and capable of changing the world. He has also directed the admission process into a law school, and found the same type of bright, driven, capable candidates. For the last seven years, he has supervised admissions to UACOM-Phoenix. He screens thousands of applicants annually, and he finds the medical school candidates to also be bright, well educated, capable, and disciplined in their approach. They want to be in charge and want to change the world. What sets them apart is they are driven to serve humanity. American medicine needs to grasp, foster, and utilize that distinction. It holds a world of potential and promise.

I use a few new terms in this book. The term "medical-industrial complex" refers to everything in the world of medicine: hospitals and hospital chains, nurses, administrations, medical colleges, residency programs, large research endeavors, healthcare insurance systems, pharmaceutical industries, including drug stores on every other street corner, and all the doctors' offices, urgent cares, and their employees. It includes all the support systems needed to keep everything running, including governmental agencies, electronic medical record systems, the various administrative employees, and medical legal endeavors. The number of entities involved in healthcare is massive and the inertia of all these activities is entrapping. When this medical legal complex becomes interwoven with profiteering that reduces the health and welfare of our populace, it may be considered structural anti-humanism. Most people involved in medical care in America are not cornerstones invested in maintaining the status quo. However, some major players such as the pharmaceutical industry, and the health insurance industry, are extremely committed to continuing the current state-of-affairs. They are the "oligarchs" of modern medicine. Physicianship refers to the full blooded, mature practice of medicine: adhering to the scientific, remembering our social values, but most importantly, keeping the welfare of the patient first.

Every fall I take a trip to Tijuana, Mexico, with a group of first and second year medical students at the UACOM- Phoenix, to provide medical attention to immigrants at our border. These students are a treat. They are bright, energetic, selfless, serious, and relaxed in the roles they divvy up. They have fun as people in their twenties do and they find meaning in this endeavor. The poverty we see is mind-boggling. But the students persevere. This is the potential and promise our modern healthcare industry is wasting.

Who in the world of medicine has more undirected potential than our beginning medical students? Our present day for-profit corporate practice of medicine directs them away from the humanistic. Our system of medical education is also at fault, by not preparing students to face the silos of medicine. The goals and values of the quadruple aim ought to be a source of discussion and research throughout the four years of medical school. Medical educators are committed individuals, parsing out the scientific truths of their fields, teaching and focusing on their academic careers. But many do not have familiarity with the realities of nonacademic medicine. They are the first models for the students, yet most medical students do not go into academics.

The students accepted into medical schools are among the top of their college peers. The competition is formidable. More than 53,000 students apply to Allopathic Medical schools annually, and in 2021, only 23,000 were admitted–an acceptance rate of 43%. [(1)] The necessary background curriculum must demonstrate excellent performance in the sciences and mathematics. Want to shake up your doctor? Ask him or her how much he enjoyed organic chemistry. That one course is a major hurdle for all medical students. They also must excel in some liberal arts field such as history, sociology, languages, etc. The volume of information is daunting. They must demonstrate that they can swallow from a fire hydrant of information. Accomplishment in some nonacademic field is expected. This could be in music, volunteer work, sports, etc. Another part of the gauntlet is studying for, taking, and being strikingly successful on the Medical College Admissions Test, the famous MCAT exam. This one exam is usually taken after college graduation, when several months of concentrated study can be devoted to preparation. Of course, strong references from employers or professors are expected. And finally, there are in-person interviews in which one must demonstrate a mature, socially appropriate presence, engaging, not overwhelming, and not obsequious.

This is the raw material, the *tabula rasa,* society presents to medical schools. By the time, they graduate four years later, they will be accomplished in the medical sciences. They are taught information at the forefront of normal human physiology, and anatomy, and they become knowledgeable in the science of pathology and disease. My daughter happens to be a second-year medical student now, and what she is currently studying certainly exceeds the knowledge base I was exposed to 46 years ago. Our ability to treat cardiovascular disease, cancer, infections, and other disease processes has improved a great deal over the last four decades. Medical students are exposed to these wonders and have opportunities to decide upon the field, where they want to spend their careers. Their further training occurs in their internships and residencies.

Interns are exposed to and inured to the stresses of the practice of medicine. On my first day on call as an intern, I was asked to see a patient with a heart rhythm problem – supraventricular tachycardia. At that time, massaging the carotid artery was standard treatment to end the rhythm, so I gently performed it. The next day he had had a stroke, which no doubt the carotid massage had caused. I felt horrible, but I learned two things: to take "standard practice" with a grain of salt. I have not performed that procedure since. And I learned that bad things happen in medicine despite your best efforts, and you have to stand back up, get in your scrubs, and see the next patient. This birth into the responsibility for illness, life, and death makes the internship year the toughest year of one's life. It was for me.

However, the students will make it through their internship and residency, and perhaps fellowship training and then assume a role somewhere in the practice of medicine. Sooner or later, their leadership potential, their own unique talents, may blossom.

All society should benefit from these best and hardest working minds, but too often the many prescribed activities from the silos of medicine prevent this maturation. The for-profit corporate practice of medicine assumes control. All that potential remains as a pawn on the chess board, played by the corporations. It is constrained in range and power. That unique combination of intelligence, drive, years of education, and desire to serve humanity is squashed by our medical industrial complex.

I have been to medical conferences on leadership. Perhaps in an effort to inject humor, a slide may be projected showing cats scrambling along and cowboys on horseback behind them. The administrative lament is that their job of controlling doctors is as difficult as "herding cats." What an insult! To compare a physician to a housecat is offensive. Much of what is wrong in medicine could be fixed if the potential of physicians and especially primary care physicians was allowed to be at play.

Consider the word "agency." Generally, we focus on the organizational sense of agency; a group of people specifically vetted and empowered by the populace to carry out certain supervisory tasks. "Agency," derives from the Medieval Latin: *agentia*, "To do, act, manage." We have come to consider agency to be a grouping of people, but the heart of this word has to do with action, with stepping forth responsibly, no matter the number of actors involved. It has to do with assessing the situation, weighing the possibilities, and consequences, and working to improve outcomes.

A friend related an event, when he was driving alone down Grand Avenue in Phoenix, a diagonal thoroughfare with only a few stoplights. The traffic was light and speeds in the sixties were common. Suddenly, a toddler staggered out the open doors of a furniture warehouse and walked into the street by himself. There was no shoulder to pull onto. My friend stopped in the lane, scooped up the child, put him in his car, and found a nearby parking lot. Soon enough the parents emerged, frantically seeking their child. My friend honked and waved and a joyous reunion ensued.

Were there considerations of accusations of kidnapping on my friend's part or child neglect by the parents? I suppose, but the catastrophic possible outcomes, and the immediacy of the situation called for action and a good outcome was achieved. There was no time for committee review, and no manual of recommendations covering this situation. No time to call the police or child protective services. Delay would have been completely irresponsible. My friend utilized his value system as a parent himself and as a socialized human being. He did the right thing. He had agency.

Heroism commonly has to do with going against the flow of group think. Martin Luther voiced the Protestant Reformation, Martin Luther King Jr., dreamed of a future with racial harmony, and Mahatma Gandhi inspired the independence of India. They all saw major wrongs and initiated action to better things. The raw courage of Sojourner Truth, the daunting creativity of Maria Montessori, and the prescience of Rachel Carson are all examples of agency. Without the idiosyncratic vision of these leaders, and their willingness to swim against the flow of group think, our global society would be far less developed.

That sense of individual agency may be expressed in a group setting. Our Supreme Court comes to mind. The individuals comprising the Court are vetted to the last degree by their education, work experience, and by our political process. The power of this very select small group of people derives from their willingness to consider the arguments thoroughly and arrive intelligently at their own opinion. Each is expected to express and vote his individual mind. Their power as a group derives from their superior individual competence and their commitment to knowing and acting on their own mind. (Our current Justices may seem to have been influenced by our political process. There is nothing new about that. From the beginning of our nation, the Supreme Court has been influenced by the social values of the day.)

Daniel Pink has written a book, *DRIVE: The Surprising Truth About What Motivates Us* (2009) This book begins by reviewing a good deal of industrial psychology. He convincingly shows that traditional carrots and sticks actually impede rather than enhance performance. Most of us assume money is the prime driver. It is important, but other factors, specifically autonomy, mastery, and purpose are of greater importance, assuming the financial impact is marginal. As it turns out, having the opportunity to determine one's own work priorities, is worth some sacrifice in income. Having the ability to become proficient in one's work, to master the work, is a major motivator. And having the sense that one is significantly helping society, to have purpose, is worth a certain margin of income. Autonomy, mastery, and purpose are all integral to agency. These are the driving forces that will prevail, <u>assuming the financial impact is minimal.</u>

I have touched on the differences of specialist physicians and primary care physicians. I would like to elaborate on these differences as they are important. First, the amount of training is greater to be a specialist. They may spend two to six years focusing on one body part, disease, or procedure. For instance, ophthalmologists are experts in eyes and vision. General ophthalmologists are becoming rare. Many ophthalmologists in training subspecialize in a single part of this important one ounce bit of flesh. Some specialize in the back of the eye, (retinologists) or in cataract procedures at the front of the eye, etc. Cardiologists can subspecialize in the impulse conduction system (electrophysiologists), or heart failure, or cardiac circulation. The upside of specialization is expertise in a smaller segment of our healthcare spectrum. The downside is the lack of general medical knowledge, and the lack of broader knowledge regarding how all the parts of our medical system fit together.

These specialists are not prepared for health problems outside of their organ system of choice, much less to address depression, or social issues such as abuse, etc. If confronted with a problem apart from their knowledge base, they are apt to instruct the patient to contact their primary care physician for a referral to another specialist. I recently had a patient whose problem was kidney stones, as found by a gastroenterologist at endoscopy (under fluoroscopy). She was told to contact me for a referral to a renal specialist and an urologist. Not knowing the background I asked her to come in for a visit and as it turned out she had never passed a kidney stone. There was no information as to what kind of stone this was or even that it was causing any problem. Much more can be said about the proper evaluation of asymptomatic stones in the pelvis of the kidney, and I am pursuing such an evaluation with her. But the management does not involve seeing any other specialist and does not involve any procedure to remove the stone. The role of the primary care physician is to bring some general medical knowledge, and common sense to the situation, which saves the patient painful procedures, and society money. Most specialists lack functional general medical knowledge.

Is there a role for specialization? Of course. This same patient may have been cured of a pancreatic cancer by a team of gastroenterologists, GI oncologists, radiation specialists, radiologists, nursing staff, support personnel, and by me, her internist who found the problem to begin with. A team effort was needed and there was no role for a "lone cowboy" in her management. But in addressing the quadruple aim, specialists in primary care medicine are much more effective than specialists in specialty medicine. Who can better orchestrate the efforts of community resources needed to address the medical aspects of population health? Who can better establish the trusting relationship with patients needed for improved patient experience? Who controls the most downstream dollars that affect the financial wellbeing of our healthcare system? In each case the primary care physician outperforms the specialist. Not so obvious is the question of physician wellbeing.

To a large extent, the further down the path of specialization one proceeds, the more prescribed, or directed the care becomes. This is especially true in the surgical subspecialties. At the other end of the training spectrum are the primary care physicians. They have the broadest scope of responsibility. They are expected to have substantial knowledge of all the organ systems, to know their own limitations, and to recognize what specialists are available, when the presenting problem is beyond their scope. Unlike the subspecialists' practice, where the next steps are relatively known and limited, in the fields of primary care medicine, the next steps are not so defined. To a great extent the patient, and their family may have strong views regarding what is wrong and what if anything should to be done. Social and religious considerations may be present. The family practitioner is dealing with 10 organ systems, with advancing and changing medical knowledge across the complete spectrum of human ages, and major variables of society's, families', and patients' opinions. The complexity is vast. The recommended next steps are debatable. Many times, the best answers are beyond the blunt scope of double blinded scientific studies, beyond religious dogma, and beyond legal imperatives. In the midst of this cacophony, there are multiple insurance plans, silos, each demanding that its own unique set of metrics be followed to document compliance with their idea of what is important this year. Frequently, especially in primary care medicine, the best answers are forged from a trusting relationship of the patient and family with a physician of unsurpassed scientific, and humanitarian inclinations.

If we are serious about healthcare reform, if we are serious about achieving the quadruple aim, we need a much larger share of medical students becoming generalists.

So why don't more medical students go into primary care medicine? First and foremost the compensation is much less. According to a 2020 JAMA Network article by Walter Hsiang, et.al. [(3)] in 2017 the average primary care physician's earnings were 62% that of specialists. In the current financial setting in the United States, going into primary care medicine requires a willingness to shoulder a financial impact that is not marginal. Given the expense of medical school, _paying off that debt definitely influences the long-term career choices. Our insistence on paying much more for procedures than for cognitive work clearly influences the career paths of medical students. The average medical student owes $350,000 at completion of medical school and the prospect of paying this off over a 25-year period rather than five years, clearly stimies their interest in primary care medicine. To fully utilize the potential of the students we recruit into medical schools, the difference in compensation of primary care physicians and specialists must end.

How is compensation determined? The American Medical Association has a Revenue Update Committee that advises the Center for Medicare and Medicaid Services about compensation, and this advice is followed closely. Note that the specialists and proceduralists in this advisory panel outnumber the primary care physicians, 18 to 4. What factors does the advisory committee take into consideration? Was extra training required to become a specialist? Usually it takes two or more years. At the end of the training this investment of time is more than fairly compensated. The committee also looks at malpractice liability as the premiums are greater for the procedural-lists. But again, this risk is more than fairly compensated by the salaries. There is no shortage of people wanting to be cardiologists, or dermatologists, or to enter other specialties, despite the increased time in training and the rising risks of malpractice suits. Those disadvantages are generously reimbursed by the compensation structure, leading to a shortage of primary care physicians.

A second reason medical students don't go into primary care medicine are issues of time. I have never seen a comparative time study, but I do know PCPs spend more hours completing uncompensated tasks than do many specialists. In my personal practice, the ratio of uncompensated phone calls to compensated visits is five-to- one. Either I return phone calls, or I pay someone to do callbacks. The commercial insurance silos expect us to spend time solving their pricing slight-of-hand for free.

Patients expect us to fill out insurance and disability forms for free. And don't get me started on the biggest time thief of all, the electronic medical records (EMRs). Somehow the federal government was all in for promoting EMRs, which did enrich the proprietary software developers, but the government is way too lax when it comes to disciplining these EMR corporations. Interoperability is difficult, and the requirements of privacy compliance continue to be increasingly complex. The excessive time required to manage patients using an EMR is the primary reason I stopped attending to my patients in hospitals.

Do not think that medical students are unaware of these inequities of time and money. Of course they know what the money and lifestyle differences are, not to mention the debt they are assuming upon completion of medical school. Their worries about paying off these loans forces many of them to walk away from primary care fields.

There are ongoing efforts in medical schools to recruit students into primary care medicine, but until CMS gets serious about pay equity, and does something to address the lifestyle issues, this problem will continue. Until the specialists who rule the AMA RUC are reigned in, pay and time inequity will persist, and medical students will continue to avoid the primary care fields. The quadruple aims will be inadequately served.

Physicians potentially have a great deal of agency. They are in or ought to be in position to accomplish much of the quadruple aim. In medical school they ought to be exposed to this framework to optimize healthcare systems. My daughter is now a third-year medical student at the UACOM-Phoenix. I recently asked her and a classmate, a combined PhD and MD candidate, about their exposure to these larger problems of our healthcare system. They have had no formal time to consider the quadruple aim. This is typical of most medical schools in the United States.

Think of it. The dismal financial performance of healthcare in the United States could be improved if medical students were made aware of our last place status among developed countries. These young and impressionable medical students would ultimately do a better job of caring for the indigent if they were exposed early in their training to the need for such care. In terms of financial performance, the U.S. is in last place. If physicians had the freedom to own and manage their own practices, to manage the time they spend with the patients, they would do a better job of assuring their patients were happy with their services. If the expected course for young doctors after completion of their formal training, were to join an independent group of doctors, all interested in their own autonomy, professionalism, and purpose, wouldn't their job satisfaction improve?

About 2,000,000 people complete undergraduate school each year. Of these people roughly 3% apply to medical schools and roughly 1%, 20,000, are accepted. One would be hard pressed to find another grouping of 20,000 in those

2 million graduates who have a greater combination of scientific abilities and humanitarian values than those medical college matriculants. Their potential for solving the major problems with American medicine, which we will next explore, is excellent. Their agency should not be focused toward the financial gain of large corporations.

A change is in order.

Chapter Four

Financial Responsibility

Today, November 6, 2022, is two days before midterm elections, and again we are all anxious to know who will win. No matter your leanings, right or left, we can all agree that saving money is a good idea. So, the first aim I would like to address is achieving financial wellbeing in healthcare. That means it is affordable for everyone and does not consume an excessive portion of our GNP. These are reasonable expectations for this wealthy and smart country of ours.

Healthcare is a huge part of our national financial picture, approaching 20% of our Gross National Product. Decidedly, in healthcare we are a huge financial failure. Many millions of people suffer, and a very few get very rich. In this chapter, I will review the facts, explore the reasons, and suggest solutions.

According to the Peterson-Kaiser Family Foundation Health Systems Tracker [(1)] among 12 nations considered to be first world, the United States ranked last in terms of per capita expense of healthcare. The best was the United Kingdom, and in descending order, Japan, Australia, France, Canada, Belgium, the Netherlands, Sweden, Austria, Germany, Switzerland, and last was the United States. In 2019, the cost of healthcare for every individual in the U.S. was $10,966. In next highest nation, Switzerland, the annual per capita cost was $7,732. The average of these 12 nations was $5,697, and the lowest, in the UK, it was $4,653. So, healthcare in America costs about twice as much as in the average nation in this comparison. In 2019 the U.S. spent $3.8 trillion, and that number goes up ~$50 billion every year.

Among first world countries by far we spend the most money. We must be getting a high quality product, right? The Commonwealth Fund is a major philanthropic organization that monitors the quality of healthcare on an ongoing basis. It regularly issues reports based on data from a variety of international organizations, including the Organization for Economic Co-operation and Development (OECD), and the Peterson-Kaiser-FF. Overall, the U.S. ranked dead last in a ranking of these top 10 wealthy nations in terms of overall healthcare. We were behind the United Kingdom, Switzerland, Sweden, Australia, Germany, the Netherlands, Norway, France, and Canada. We have the lowest life expectancy, the highest maternal and newborn mortality rate, the highest suicide rate, the highest chronic disease burden, the highest obesity rate, the fewest per capita physicians, and the highest rate of hospitalizations for preventable causes.

We are behind, not by a little, but a lot. It would be reasonable to ask if there is anything those countries are doing that we are not. Why is the U.S., such an outlier? There is an answer. It is that those other countries, save the Netherlands, all have single-payor healthcare. The Netherlands has multiple payors, but the terms and benefits are all highly defined. The King Kong in the U.S. system, that we are all controlled by, is the fiction, the lie, that if we moved to a single-payor system, it would be a slippery slope into communistic socialism.

The largest payor of healthcare in the U.S., is the Center for Medicare and Medicaid Services (CMS.) Each year it produces a report called the National Health Expenditure Data (NHED) [(3)], which reviews our financial performance dating back to 1960, and projecting ahead to 2028. In case you are wondering, CMS has an Office of Actuary, which publishes an analysis of these projections. Bottom line, they get it right to within 1% year after year.

Per this NHED report in 1960, healthcare expenses were 5% of the GNP in the United States. Our total national medical expense was $27.2 billion, and our per capita expense was $146. In 2020 healthcare was over $4.01 trillion, it was 18% of our GNP, at a cost of $12,118 per individual. For every man, woman, and child, our healthcare costs us more than $12,000 per year. Healthcare expense in the United States has gone up dramatically. Someone has kept his foot on the gas pedal.

Just how did we get to this point? Many of the mechanisms to be covered here have already been well addressed by Marty Makary, MD in his book, *The Price We Pay*, 2019. (4) His writing style is engaging and he addresses many of the unfair and wasteful practices in our healthcare. Other sources are from the medical literature, especially from the JAMA.

An important study was published in JAMA in 2017 by Dr. Joseph Dieleman PhD, (5) addressing the components of healthcare spending increases between 1996 at $1.2 trillion and 2013 at $2.1 trillion. Population growth went up by 23% and aging of the population by 12%. We cannot do much about these factors. Disease prevalence actually decreased by 2.4%. Changes in service utilization was not significantly changed. Pricing of services and intensity of services went up by 50% between 1996 and 2013. Obviously, our focus needs to be on the prices we charge for various services and treatments, and the number of services and treatments we arrange for each episode of illness, be it acute or chronic. These are the factors that explain why healthcare debt is the major cause of bankruptcy in the US, and it explains our loser status regarding our healthcare expense among first world nations.

There are many mechanisms by which pricing and intensity of services are increased. Again, many of these practices have been exposed by multiple experts in healthcare financing, including Dr. Makary, by Mr. Wendell Potter, in *Deadly Spin* and by many academics, such as Dr. Dieleman.

Let's track the healthcare financial experience of Ms. Sarah Doe. Money is very tight for this 32-year-old single mother of two small children, Linda, 7, and Jack, 5. Sarah works as an administrative assistant in the large Home Delivery Corporation (HDC). Sarah was shocked at the cost, when it came time to select a health insurance plan. The minimum hourly wage in New York State is $12.25 per hour. This works out to $25,000 per year or about $1000 per paycheck. The minimum wage goes down in most other states. Out of that money she pays taxes, provides shelter, food, clothing, and transportation for herself, and Linda and Jack. She settled on an insurance plan from Care a Lot Health. In this plan, she will be able to somewhat afford monthly premiums which will cover routine doctor visits after the deductible has been met, but requires a very large co-pay for major problems. Her monthly premiums will be

$200, and she has a deductible of $7,500, to meet if she or her children encounter a major health event.

Note that many of Sarah's peers choose to go bare. They have no insurance. If there is a minor problem they will pay cash at the local urgent care. If there is a major problem, if hospitalization is required, bankruptcy lies right ahead.

Why are Care a Lot premiums so high? They are faced with escalating doctor, hospital, and pharmaceutical costs. They also are faced with advertising budgets, which are necessary to remain competitive. Remember, competition is a good thing. They also must pay their high-priced corner suite administration at salaries Sarah Doe would find unfathomable. To justify their earnings, these top administrators must create profits to pass along to their stockholders. Also, the major healthcare insurance companies all must pay their dues to the shell corporations, they create by colluding with their "competitors" to lobby our elected representatives, and dupe the public to maintain the illusion of free competition. Please see Potter's *Deadly Spin* for a well-documented expose'. These front groups all have warm inviting names like Coalition for Affordable Healthcare, Health Benefits Corporation, and America's Health Insurance Plans. They aim to maintain the status quo. First in expense, last in quality.

All of these expenses bear down on Care a Lot and they pass that expense along to their individual customers, and to the employers of those customers. That expense does dig into the salaries HDC is able to pay its employees. Raises are out of the question because those potential funds are used for healthcare inflation.

Sarah took the kids to visit their grandparents. On the way home, there was a serious car accident, and Linda was severely injured with a fractured femur. Several emergency helicopters were immediately on the scene. Emergency transport is a very lucrative business. It can be unscrupulous. In years past, helicopter emergency transport was managed by not-for-profit hospitals and the bills were reasonable, and submitted to the insurance companies, and as part of the hospital tab. Over the past few decades, this service has been outsourced to private concerns. They are at liberty to charge whatever they please. Bills are common in the $20,000 to $50,000 range and up. And commonly the patients who are transported actually have no emergency at all. As for

Sarah, she received a bill for $25,000, for Linda's helicopter ride. She had no financial reserves to pay this bill. The insurance companies no longer cover this service, because it is not part of a hospital bill. Each of the doctors involved in the care, the surgeon, anesthesiologist, hospitalist, emergency room doctor, and the radiologist each submitted separate bills to her. The total of the doctors' billing was $10,000, which was elevated because there were no negotiated in-network discounts. The hospital's bill, which included the operative facility fee, was $75,000. Sarah's expenses were now well over $100,000. She had to file for bankruptcy because she did not have the money for even the deductible, and that ended her hopes for a future college education.

This has been a tour of the financial debacle perpetrated by our healthcare system. This family was imaginary, but their financial experience was not in the least imaginary. It is experienced by thousands of Americans daily. Again, healthcare expense is the most common cause of bankruptcy in the United States. This debacle is perpetuated by our for- profit corporations running our healthcare system.

Now imagine if we had a single-payor healthcare system. The cost of the helicopter ride would be negotiated and because this transport business was coordinated, only one helicopter would have been dispatched. There would be no out-of-network surprise billing from the doctors and the hospital. In many countries listed previously, there would have been no charge at all to the family. And in those countries the total healthcare expense is less and the overall quality is superior to that of the United States. A single- payor healthcare system is widely acknowledged as the direction we should pursue. Many of the corporations that manage our healthcare system do very well.

Milton Friedman, the economist, would be proud. But the profits of a few at the expense of the many does not equal economic well-being. Each of the quadruple aims, affordability, population health, patient experience in healthcare, and physician well-being are separate issues. But the problems all of them are having, I lay directly at the feet of the oligarch corporate practice of medicine. I believe the solution to these problems lies, in the short run, in the hands of our elected leaders, and longer term in the hand of our physicians to be.

That a few major healthcare insurers can coalesce into nice sounding front groups, hiding their anonymity, is suspicious. That these groups contribute millions to our congressional leaders is more than suspicious, and that the laws these leaders pass always fall to the benefit of these commercial companies is outrageous.

One of the issues that continues to come up is that each individual aim can interfere with the other aims. Putting physician well-being first can have negative consequences on patient experience, population health, and financial well- being. When an institution puts financial success first, it is unlikely to be doing its fair share for population health, physician well-being, and patient experience. Some highly regarded hospital systems refuse to accept standard Medicare or Medicaid reimbursement rates. Full payment is expected for all services. Perhaps such systems should not be so highly regarded. That is, any rating experts should consider all aspects of healthcare, including affordability for the indigent, prior to handing out accolades.

How do we start to change our financial embarrassment? First, we have to recognize that there is a problem. Anyone with any knowledge about healthcare understands, there is a problem. The facts presented earlier in this chapter have been known by many for years and are repeated here for the uninitiated. Everyone in America should have a passing awareness of these healthcare issues. Many already know medical care in America is very expensive. They should also know how little we get for those dollars. This largely falls on our formal media and on our social media. Change is needed and it is coming, needed or not. Medicare will be bankrupt in two more years, and a major review of healthcare in America will occur.

Second, we need to encourage our medical students to become aware of healthcare social issues. My recollection of medical education is that it consists of a deluge of factoids, some important and many not. Dr. Makary is hilarious in describing how many times he has learned and forgotten the details of the Krebs cycle (the ten different biochemical steps need to produce our energy.) Perhaps the problem is rooted in the academic totem of our medical schools. Terms like students, tests, college, tenure, professors, and departmental chairs all derive from academia. Commonly, medical professors do not have a clue about the real world problems their students are about to face, as these problems are a result of the business world. Given the importance of the quadruple aim, substantial time in medical school should be committed to its study, as it is much more important than the Krebs cycle. Our future leaders need to explore the basic issues of the quadruple aim. I do not say they should be instructed in the quadruple aim as no one has all the answers yet. Akin to laying down railroad track, while the healthcare train is hurtling into the future, our bright, and humanistic medical students need to explore, and create changes themselves. There is no doubt that these medical students will graduate from medical school, they will succeed in their residencies and fellowships, and they will begin to practice medicine. At some point they will have a choice of following along on the treadmill of the medical-industrial complex, permitting the MBAs to lead the way. Or, if properly aware of these financial problems, and of their cachet, power, and agency, they can begin to forge a new future for healthcare in America.

Third, our elected leaders need to be aware of these issues. They need to be stout in governing the medical- industrial complex, our corporate oligarchs, and they need to be forceful in creating a path to a universal payor system. I believe that we need a trail of half-steps because of the size of our current system, its variability, and its complicated entrenchment in our economy. That trail will likely include a "public option" which is already being tried in several states.

It is tempting to point fingers. Some people argue that everyone should have a "right" to healthcare. I disagree with this as "rights" are defined by our Constitution in the Bill of Rights, and in the first 10 amendments. However, I do think everyone "ought" to have healthcare. By far, most people agree with this. If most people did not agree with this, we would not have ambulances and emergency rooms and we would see people dying on the streets. The problem is that emergency rooms are a terribly expensive, and dysfunctional system to care for uninsured people.

I think healthcare is best thought of as a utility, like electricity and water, and like the police department and the fire department. It would be inappropriate to own shares in a fire department, expecting a return on the investment if the fires of the wealthy were extinguished, and ignoring the fires of people who could not afford to pay for the service. This consideration begins to get at why healthcare is a special financial case. Like water, healthcare is a fundamental need. Unlike water, the provision of healthcare is education, people and systems intensive, and therefore a lot of money is moving around. This gives rise to the entry of for-profit corporations in the U.S. into the practice of medicine. The profit motive can bring about unethical medical decisions. To get past this stage, American healthcare needs to evolve into a single-payor system.

We, the people of the United States, deserve better.

Chapter Five
Physician Well-Being

Three days ago, my daughter, now a third year medical student, told me that one of her classmates had just died of an overdose of alcohol and Xanax. He was an excellent student, and well liked, but the stress of medical school became too great of a burden. The students in his class, and the entire faculty, including the Dean of Admissions mentioned in the Agency chapter, were in tears at the memorial service. They felt that dreadful emptiness of a premature death. Those who knew him well, felt the wind in their sails, the charge of medical school, drop away.

The stress of medicine has always been with us. Forty- five years ago, right after graduation, one of my classmates committed suicide. He had been accepted into a prestigious surgical program in Boston. The word was that he feared he could not stand up to the expectations of that program. I did not know him well. Medical students often run in packs and we were not in the same group of friends. I do remember, he was rather quiet, concerned, and ethical, obviously talented, and he, like the most of us, had worked hard to press through medical school in three years. I recall feeling that the loss was stunning, both for his family, and classmates on a personal level, and for our society as a whole. That potential to be a strong surgeon, the intelligence, the many years of work to obtain a topflight education, were all voided.

Certainly, there is a sheen to being a physician, which the public may respect or resent. Please understand that there is a dark side of pressure, which all doctors will learn to manage, in ways healthy or unhealthy. The same is true for others in medicine such as nurses, nurse practitioners, physician assistants, and other decision makers. We know this dark side as burnout. According to the National Academy of Medicine, burnout is "a workplace syndrome characterized by emotional exhaustion, high depersonalization (i.e. cynicism), and a low sense of personal accomplishment from work."

I experienced burnout in 1999, after shifting from the traditional role of caring for my patients both in the office and in the hospital, to being a hospitalist, a doctor who only works in hospitals. Their task is to process the patients through as rapidly as possible, which saves the hospitals money, as their reimbursement is now based on the average care deemed necessary for the admitting diagnosis, not by the number of days the patient actually remains in the hospital. My workmates and I covered the entire Phoenix metropolitan area, which is 100 miles across, seeing patients in a variety of hospitals. There was no follow-up and no closure with these patients. This was not at all what I do best. Mixed in with this burnout, I became depressed, a heavy and deeply hopeless feeling. Every morning, was a dark burden. I hate to quit any project, but there was my family and my own happiness to consider, so I resigned from that hospitalist position, and saw a psychiatrist who started me on Prozac. I felt the curtain beginning to lift at three weeks and the joy of hope returned. Four weeks later I was back at my previous job and life was good again.

I have been fully open in revealing my history of depression and there has never been any recrimination from our state medical board, from my colleagues, or from my patients. When I prescribe antidepressants to my patients, I always reveal that I take them myself. Some of the most fulfilling experiences I have had were helping depressed men and women through their depression. I have never again been as depressed as in 1999. I take these medications now to help keep my anger under reign. As we are seeing, there are plenty of reasons to be angry about healthcare.

There are just over 1,000,000 practicing physicians in the U.S. and every year we lose between 300 and 400 to suicide, twice the rate of the general population. Clearly burnout and depression contribute to this suicide rate. Interestingly, at matriculation into medical school, these students have above average mental health. A 2022 survey of 9175, physicians, representing all states, and most specialties, published by Medscape, gives further detail. Fifty-three percent of physicians said, they were burned out, and 23% reported depression, both statistics higher than five years ago. The highest rates were found in doctors practicing emergency medicine, in internal medicine, and in pediatrics. The lowest rates were in pathology and public health. The most commonly cited reason for burnout was excessive bureaucratic demands. Females suffered burnout at a 63% rate, and males at 53%. (And women have a higher suicide rate.) Sixty-five percent of respondents said, their work had a negative impact on their relationships.

The work setting made a difference. The most burnout was found in multispecialty practices, at 57%. And, the least was in office-based solo practices, at 43%. An anonymous telling quote adds a human touch. "Only a sociopath could practice as an employee of a large health system and not be burned out. Anyone who cares about patients is doomed to burnout."

Certainly, stress and depression do not lead to suicide attempts in most cases, but it is well documented that it detracts from one's performance in other ways. As one's attitude declines it may lead to decreasing one's workload. Even if the hours are not reduced, it commonly affects the quality of the care given. As pressures mount, a geographic escape is common. Leaving one company and landing elsewhere is another form of escape. The burnout may lead to quitting the practice of medicine entirely. That is, after accumulating $300,000 to $400,000 of debt for medical school, after spending seven to ten years or more in training, after establishing relationships with patients and coworkers, the atmosphere, and outlook is so bleak it is not worth continuing. Since the pandemic began, roughly 18% of healthcare workers have left the field.

Burnout has its costs beyond the personal. There are financial losses to the company. Dr. Tate Shanafelt, who is recognized nationally as an authority on healthcare burnout, has written extensively about the financial cost of replacing a physician in a large corporation. Between lost revenue, recruiting costs of a replacement, startup expenses, the average financial expense for replacing a specialty physician ranges from $500,000 to 1 million dollars. Why is burnout so prevalent? An overview comes from a report of the National Academy of Medicine. [(1)] "Humanism and professionalism are two major motivating factors for most clinicians, and many aspects of the modern work environment conflict with these fundamental ethical norms. Regulatory and institutional policies, payer requirements, and intrusive, difficult technologies all challenge the basic ethical motivations that are essential to professional fulfillment of the human beings who are central to high- quality patient care."

The time and stress demands have been widely recognized since modern medicine began. What does it take to thrive under these circumstances? Beginning to describe a successful path is a 2019 article in Health Affairs by Dr. Samuel Edwards, et. al,

"Cultural and Structural Features of Zero-Burnout Primary Care Practices." They analyzed the findings from a survey by the Agency for Healthcare Research and Quality. Of 715 primary care practices in the United States, one-third had no burnout at all, but one-fifth of the groups had 40% or more of physicians burned out. How did they differ?

Seven times in this article, the word agency is used as a positive feature, as in "agency is a protective factor for organizational and professional well-being." Smaller practices, solo practices, and clinician owned practices, had less burnout. Those practices not participating in demonstration projects such as accountable care organizations (in which external rather than internal input for improvement is greater) had less burnout. Also, the more successful practices had facilitative leadership, which promoted an environment in which things can be accomplished; people at all levels could openly talk about what is and isn't working, and people had an opportunity to grow in their work. An eye opener is what did not make a difference. Changes in electronic health records, loss of clinicians, number of patients seen by each provider per day, and the proportion of Medicaid patients seen, did not differentiate.

What is really going on here? *The American Journal of Medicine*, Sept 2021, contains a starting place in an article by Dr. Steven Southwick, et. al. (6) "Rediscovering Meaning and Purpose: An Approach to Burnout in the Time of COVID-19 and Beyond." He cites Dr. Victor Frankle's fascinating book, *Man's Search for Meaning*, 1959. (7) Dr. Frankle, was the MD psychiatrist who, through spirit and determination, endured three years in a Nazi concentration camp. In his book, he details the human degradation, the starvation, and the constant threat of death. Upon arrival, the prisoners were separated from all family, stripped of all clothing and shaved of all hair. Repeatedly his life was at stake. Using hard work, his psychiatric training, and his smarts, he managed to survive. Many of his fellow prisoners became completely numb to the horror, gave up hope, and soon died. For Dr. Frankle, staying alive while surrounded by death, became a victory, a purpose and meaning in itself. Out of this experience he founded an entire school of psychiatric thought, Logotherapy. "Man's search for meaning is the prime motivation in his life and not a "secondary rationalization" of instinctual drives. This meaning is unique and specific in that it must and can be fulfilled by him alone; only then does it achieve a significance which will satisfy his own will to meaning." (7) Dr. Southwick's article points toward a recent survey of 2000 members of the American Academy of Family Physicians. "The factor most strongly associated with physician happiness was career purpose, which includes satisfaction, joy in work, spiritual purpose, and meaningful patient relationships. A sense of calling and having long-term relationships with patients were strongly associated with high life meaning. In most cases, extrinsic motivators, such as annual income or other work-related characteristics, were not related to well-being, life satisfaction, life meaning, or career commitment." (6)

An important shift occurred in medicine's view of burnout over the last 30 years. Initially, companies losing revenue due to burnout blamed individual physicians being unable to cope with their workload. The physician was the element needing to be changed. Wellness tactics including detailed instructions on meditation and yoga, increased time off, and reorganization of their workload were attempted, and failed. Burnout continued to grow. More recently it became apparent that the problem lay within the organization itself. A major 2019 report from the National Academy of Medicine, "Taking Action Against

Clinician Burnout: A Systems Approach to Professional Wellbeing" pointed to evidence that, unshackled, the physicians were capable of handling large workloads and weathering other stressors that occur when caring for people with major health problems.

Daniel Pink wrote *Drive: The Surprising Truth About What Motivates Us,* 2009. [8] This fascinating book argues that our main motivators are not financial, or other perks that are associated with top performance in the business world. There is little benefit from punishments. He shows that punishments only get in the way. He shows us that top performance is associated with three factors: autonomy, mastery, and purpose. Of course, a reasonably competitive salary and the usual acknowledgements of status are important, but if present, they are only a necessary foundation and rarely increase individual physician performance.

Pink's arguments are based on animal experiments and studies of human behavior. These studies are a continuation of the work in the field of behavioral economics, which earned Daniel Kahneman a Nobel Prize in 2002. The conclusion of *Drive* shows that it takes more than a strict calculation of profitability to govern one's behavior. Pink reviews long established demonstrations that raisins and money do not reliably control the performance of monkeys, and college freshmen. In fact, dangling such rewards only interferes with achievement.

Autonomy to choose one's own schedules, tasks, technique, and workmates enhances performance. Multiple studies from the business world demonstrate this. "We're meant to be players, not pawns… But outside forces, including the very idea that we need to be "managed" have conspired to change our default setting…." (8) Premed students in college and afterwards drive themselves with impressive intrinsic motivation. They are selected into medical schools because their talent and iron show through. They are forged by training into steel. Upon completing their training, they are ready to put their agency to work. The floundering and confusing mandates of the multiple silos can undermine this agency. Their narrow financial goals miss the aim of improving the physician experience by a long shot.

Mastery is another prime motivator. In major industrial studies, it has been demonstrated that the urge to master new and engaging work is the best predictor of productivity. It beats financial incentives. Hard work and long hours are a necessary part of mastery. These conditions are the life of the physician. When physicians are permitted to choose and own their work, (i.e., to become the masters of their work), they are fulfilled.

Pink's third motivator is purpose. He points toward many examples of how having a greater, more altruistic goal in life, makes for more happiness. College graduates who professed to primarily altruistic goals, prior to graduation are more satisfied with their careers than those seeking self- aggrandizement. He cites Dr. Tate Shanafelt's research at the Mayo Clinic. "Letting doctors pursue activities that were personally meaningful to them for 20% of their time, led to less than half the burnout compared to the controls.

Recall our third chapter, agency. Some people in college may choose to pursue a career in medicine. A spark of self- recognition somehow engenders this choice. It is a private decision. As a first step, they assess what it will take to get into a medical college. Then begins the alone hours of work necessary to achieve an impressive grade point average, and an exceptional score on the MCAT. This effort builds a familiarity with the scientific foundations upon which our practices rest and it demonstrates how well the candidates function under the workload they are about to experience. Can they drink and assimilate from the fire hydrant? If admitted, they face four years of medical school in which the day-to-day stress and responsibility continue to increase. Then begins an internship year, and then, residency and perhaps fellowships, all of this training lasting from three to ten years.

These are the formative experiences of the individuals who become physicians. They have earned the right to autonomy, mastery, and pursuit of their meaning and purposes, which are the building blocks of agency. Finally, they leave their training, and must decide whether to follow the traditional track the system lays out, or one of independence. The easiest path for a young doctor, is to become an employee of a large corporation, where their personal agency is of very little consequence. Office space, employment, phones, and computer issues are handled by administration. They are not controlled by the provider. They have healthcare insurance and malpractice insurance provided. Management will keep their eye on the bottom line. The turnkey solution of being an employed physician can be attractive, especially to people just completing their training. However, there are dangers along this route. If the physician or clinic does not create enough revenue, management can push people to work harder, and see more patients. If the finances do not improve, the MBAs in charge have several options: merge the clinic with another group, change locations or fire "under-producing doctors." You can always hire more management to run things. It is the nature of administration to aggrandize its responsibilities and the number of people supervised. If upper management is still unhappy with the performance, abandon the patients, the physicians, and other employees. Upper management will do whatever is necessary to protect the bottom line and the earnings of shareholders. Remember Friedman's doctrine regarding the primary obligation of management: make money for the owners of the company.

All of these maneuvers can and do happen regularly in the for-profit corporate practice of medicine.

Drs. Wendy Dean and Simon Talbot have reframed these conflicts as "moral injury." (9) They reference Daniel Pink in their multiple writings, which began in 2018. "Burnout is the end stage of accumulative moral injury generally defined as perpetrating, failure to prevent, bearing witness to, or learning about acts that transgress deeply held moral beliefs and expectations. This concept better describes (than burnout) the untenable double and triple binds that physicians are finding themselves in, whereby the countless roles, they are expected to undertake often places them in conflict with their primary moral imperative: taking care of the patient." Moral injury has become a major criticism of many other parts of our modern world as well as healthcare.

People work hard to become physicians, nurse practitioners, physician assistants, and other providers of healthcare. They work hard to maintain their education. They deserve to find fulfillment. When they relinquish control to others, especially to administrators or medical directors in corporations whose primary goal is to return a profit to their stockholders, they are more apt to have second thoughts, and to experience burnout. The implication here is radical. The medical industrial complex has got to let go.

There is a medical-industrial complex. Twenty percent of the dollars in America are spent on this complex. As we have abundantly seen, this system is twice as expensive as it needs to be. The quality of our healthcare is poor. Many people in our society are left out of the system entirely. And this system is driving away many talented and committed physicians, nurses, and other medical personnel. Isn't it time for a change?

Again, healthcare should be considered a service utility. Somehow, there is a notion that it is appropriate to harness medical care for the production of profits for corporations and their shareholders. It is the dogma of the medical- industrial complex. This notion is inappropriate, but it certainly has a foothold in American medicine. It is immoral because it steps on people. The line between prudent management of resources and inappropriate denial of necessary services is too narrow for the profit motive to interfere in the judgement. For a fundamental change in thinking to take hold it will require a groundswell of opposition from the general public, and from our governmental leaders, but first we physicians must take the lead. We must find the courage to see, speak, and act on this problem. We are not cats to be herded by administrators. We must use our agency to reassert the original purposes we had as medical students, caring for people and serving humanity.

To our young physicians, it is indeed possible to find success, not only as a solo practitioner of medicine but also in small privately owned group practices. Your specialty may require you to join a larger group, but you still deserve to have a voice. Providers entering primary care medicine, which controls a major amount of downstream spending, (via testing, referrals, and hospital admissions) may be attractive targets for the for-profit corporations. You do not have to play along. Please take time to explore all your options. Think about the long run. Private practice may be the more difficult road initially, but in the long run it will leave you in control and happier.

The notion of going on your own may be intimidating, but you had what it takes to make it into and through medical school, your residency, and possibly through a fellowship. You have a lot going for you. There are many experts, accountants, real estate agents, business advisors, billing agencies, attorneys, family members, etc. who can help along the way. I am not a strong businessman, but when I started my private practice in 1981, I was amazed at how everything fell in place upon my taking out a small loan, and declaring my intention to start that practice.

Keep your agency.

Chapter Six

Patient Experience

Two years ago, we underwent an insurrection at the United States Capitol by a mob, trying to disrupt the election of the previous fall. Last year I wrote that we had weathered the storm. Today, I am not so sure. That event, somehow amalgamated with the Covid pandemic (now the omicron variant), continues to divide us, the American people, deeply. That division captures a great deal of attention. The problems that I address in this book affect all of us, right and left, and the solutions I promote can benefit us all. All of us are subject to the negative lottery of healthcare misadventures. We all want competent physicians around when an elderly parent or a child is sick. Few of us would really want to see people dying on the streets without any medical attention. Most all of us want doctors who are caring. I have many patients who scoff at the Covid vaccines, which I do endorse, but they do come to me for advice when there is a medical crisis. Healthcare spans the political divide.

Two weekends ago, I was at a reunion of my undergraduate classmates. (Our graduation was in 1971.) Soon the conversation turned to healthcare, as it commonly does. In sharp words and terse sentences, the failings of the modern healthcare system were made more than clear. Medical care is too expensive, and it is difficult to get appointments with most doctors. Care is impersonal, hurried, and time for questions is not provided. Some doctors, not all, are as seen as arrogant. American medicine can be great when you have a more serious condition. The delivery of routine care falters.

Of the four aims, patient experience is the most subjective and least quantifiable. It is easy to find quantitative information about healthcare expense, physician burnout, and public health issues. Articles are published in the medical literature presenting findings from controlled, double-blinded studies, or statistical reviews of patient populations. While relatively objective, these areas have simple a priori assumptions. Most would agree that healthcare is too expensive, that physicians leaving practice prematurely is not a good thing and that all people in our society ought to have adequate healthcare. Such underpinning assumptions cannot be made regarding the desirable patient experience. Widely differing desiderata pop up. Does the patient want to encounter a caring provider, or a broadly knowledgeable doctor, or a crisp and timely in- and-out visit? The literature on patient experience is more opinion based.

Semantics are important here. In the past we have referred to this area as "patient satisfaction." The distinction between patient experience and satisfaction has been elaborated by the NIH's Agency for Healthcare Research and Quality. [(1)] This distinction explains some of the quantification difficulty. Patient satisfaction has to do with the extent to which, expectations are being met, and these expectations are quite subjective and variable from patient to patient. This variability in expectations gives rise to differing levels of patient satisfaction for the identical management of an identical problem by the same physician. On the other hand, patient experience has much less variability. How long did you have to wait to see the physician? Were you given a chance to ask questions? Did the support staff handle the referrals, testing, and prescriptions expertly? These questions address the actual experience of healthcare in a more objective fashion, giving rise to more reliable assessments.

The most reliable and well-designed resource on patient experience comes from an agency of the United States Department of Health and Human Services (HHS). HHS directs 11 different agencies, including the Food and Drug Administration, the Center for Disease Control, the National Institute of Health, and the Centers for Medicare and Medicaid Services. Among these 11 is the Agency for Healthcare Research and Quality (AHRQ). The mission of AHRQ is to produce reliable evidence in the healthcare arena, including research into the quality of healthcare systems and frontline practitioners. To this end since 1995, they have used a survey called the Consumer Assessment of Healthcare Providers and Systems (CAHPS.) The CAHPS surveys are the gold standard of patient experience and most frequently cited in healthcare literature. Different organizations in healthcare most commonly use the CAHPS surveys to monitor and compare their performance.

So how are we doing? The nationwide CAHPS survey in 2019 [(2)] measured how frequently a top score of "good or great" was given. In terms of timeliness of appointments, we scored 65%. Our communications rated 85%. Our office staffs got a 79% for helpfulness, and we providers also got a 79% rating from our patients. Again, this is an averaging of results from many practices across the nation. I personally judge these results to be middling, not in the 90s where we can be more comfortable. While the CAHPS survey does paint with a broad brush, it does provide meaningful data. One of the architects of this survey is Rebecca Anhang Price. [(3)] "Among dozens of studies examined in a recent systematic review, the vast majority found either positive or null associations between patient experiences and best clinical practices, lower hospital readmissions, and desirable clinical outcomes."

In my review of the nongovernmental literature, I found two companies with extensive presence. The Relias Company is a subsidiary of the German conglomerate, Bertelsmann. It is a for-profit company that sells training and staff support aimed at improving the patient experience to healthcare companies such as hospitals. Their work is largely at the corporate level. They advocate the use of digital technology and the creation of patient advocacy positions within these organizations. Though all of this falls under the purview of the administrative offices, ultimately Relias does have to acknowledge the importance of the patient-provider bond.

"At the center of healthcare, however, is the healing relationship between provider and patient, a special relationship that sets healthcare apart from many other consumer driven industries… The fundamentals of creating outstanding patient experiences, lies in the cultivation of these healing relationships."

The MBAs may understand this at one level. Paint by the number guidelines can be created. But the fulfilling art of medicine will lie in the hands of authentic providers acting with agency. A December 2020 article in JAMA by Dr. Druv Khullar. (5) "Patient Consumerism, Healing Relationships, and Rebuilding Trust in Healthcare," captures a common thread in optimizing patient experience. Improving trust "starts with recognizing that despite technological, economic, and political change, trust in healthcare fundamentally begins where it always has: with healing relationships between patients and physicians."

Another major company dealing with patient experience is the non-profit Beryl Institute. It is committed to empirical research and publication of their findings. Its CEO, Jason Wolf, has published a white paper, "Consumer Perspective on Patient Experience, 2018" with a follow-up paper dated 2020. To determine just what matters to people in the healthcare world, surveys were sent to 2000 people in five countries - the U.S., Canada, the United Kingdom, the Philippines, and Australia. One finding that is not so intuitive is that, there was little variance in the values among people across these countries. Also, there was little variance across age groups.

A synopsis of the Beryl findings follows. People do care about their healthcare experience. Ninety-one percent of respondents felt it was very (32%) or extremely (59%) important. When asked what aspects of healthcare delivery were important, 56% felt the individuals they dealt with were most important. Forty-eight percent thought the process of receiving care was most important. People want to know their physical needs are being taken seriously. People want to be treated with respect and to be treated as a person, not a symptom or a diagnosis. To a relatively lesser degree people want to have a great customer experience. The costs, the parking, the food, and the building are important, but less so than the ultimate health outcome and the humanity shown in the delivery.

Who is influenced by the patients' healthcare experiences? Beryl's "Consumer Perspectives" further elaborates that the word of those experiences, good or bad, gets spread. Seventy- six percent of patients with negative experiences shared their experience, which is commonly known in the industry. What was a surprising finding is that 70% of the patients with positive experiences also share it with others. And the effects of this word of mouth are huge. In deciding where to go for healthcare, 72% of people rely on the recommendations of family and friends. Seventy percent rely on the recommendations of physicians. More formal ratings such as published rankings, awards, social media, and ratings on Yelp are considered important to less than 30% of patients.

In a summary statement, the Beryl Consumer Perspectives points away from the corporate perspective and toward the human. "Ultimately, the top identified items for consumers were about the interactions they have with people, but they are not simple interactions, they are interactions ascribed with values, the values of listening, communicating effectively, and treating others with courtesy and respect."

I write now on March 12, 2022. We all, the whole world, are watching as Russia invades, bombs and attempts to abolish the nation of Ukraine. Russia would provide top- down authoritarianism to replace the liberty of bottom-up individual agency. We should all consider the privilege and potential of using our own hard-won agency.

The CAHPS data, and the findings of Relias, and the Beryl Institute give us important data. Again and again we see that healthcare is not just another financial transaction. The literature addressing patient satisfaction is rich and gets at some important truths, which we ought not to ignore. It may be somewhat superficial, but it touches on a lot of hurt, at times rage, and it is our job to deal with it. Now, we must delve deeper.

Trust is the priceless and the most important element of the patients' experience, in healthcare. Patients and their families are dealing with unfamiliar territory with much disparate information from social media and the internet and from their many would-be experts pointing them in different directions. In the face of this confusion, getting the path right "as if your life depends on it" is not an exaggeration. Again Dr. Khullar. "A core dimension of the healthcare specific decline in trust, is a growing disconnect between what patients want and need, and what they see and experience. It is a disconnect between a transparent and trustworthy system that treats patients as humans in need of care and what many perceive as an increasingly consolidated, rofit-driven system that treats patients as consumers buying goods and services."

One of my most challenging patients ever was a 35- year-old man whose mother, a hospital administrator, asked me to see. His problem was abdominal pain, longstanding. He came to the office with most of his body covered with tattoos. He was rather thin and of medium height. He seethed in anger at the world in general and at his previous medical treatment in particular. His mother related a history of his being rendered comatose in a psychiatric ward, in an attempt to control his behavior. She checked him out of that ward once he woke up. For several years under my care he refused any psychiatric medications. He had been involved in gangs and gotten into a lot of fights in younger years. He said he was an unflinching fighter when provoked, despite his size. Previous doctors had dismissed him after a visit or two, in part because their solutions did not work, and in part because of his tattoos and attitude.

My first step was to reassure him that I would not abandon him, no matter what. Also, I had to take time to listen. The first three visits lasted an hour each and ultimately, he came to believe, I would not end my involvement, despite his vitriol, and that I would work with him and believe him. With time he started working with me and my ideas.

His chief complaint was of abdominal pain. I could not approach touching his abdomen without grimacing pain. Multiple previous evaluations, colonoscopy under sedation, and abdominal CT scans had been normal. His mother mentioned a peculiar fact. Even as a young child there were bowel problems. On a plane flight, he would spend the entire trip in a restroom. This caught my attention because while gastrointestinal disease is prone to worsening with stress, that it began in childhood pointed toward an organic cause.

We pursued extensive evaluations, and tried a variety of medications, and ultimately a variety of procedures. Under my constant supervision, he was referred to a number of chosen specialists. Surprisingly, there was no narcotic seeking behavior, though his pain continued to worsen. He did make frequent trips to emergency rooms when the pain was insurmountable, and usually he found the care there dismissive. This pattern went on for several years. During this time, I reassured him, I would never quit his case. He did not miss appointments. Trust was gradually established.

The breakthrough came with a stool marker study. The transit time of food in the colon was much longer than normal and the stools had always come out hard and painfully. He had an abnormality similar to Hirschsprung's disease, in which the nervous system in the colon fails to develop normally. This diagnosis is usually made in childhood. Ultimately, most of his colon was removed surgically and his chronic pain finally ended. He has been able to resume a normal life. He is now working as an electrician at a large construction site, his bitter past left behind.

I relate this account to emphasize the importance of trust in a patient physician-relationship. A great deal of detail and misadventures have been left out of this history. I saw him for roughly three years before a surgical cure was achieved. I did not rush him through visits. I did not discount his opinions, though they may not have been my opinions at all. With time his anger resolved, and he was able to listen to some hard truths about his situation. A correct diagnosis was achieved and a normal life restored.

Having a trusted guide is of paramount importance. What creates trust?

The medical knowledge base is a key element of trust. As one of my predecessors used to say, the kindest act a physician can perform is to make a correct diagnosis. In the face of today's explosion of information, it is impossible for any one person to keep up with everything. The use of factual resources, such as "Up to Date," (an online source of continuously updated Medical information), Epocrates for basic understanding of new medications and interactions, and the internet to investigate new findings and review old medical science, permits a real time extension of one's knowledge. Medical journals provide a wealth of ideas and knowledge. In this world of teamwork, having trusted consultants helps greatly to extend one's working knowledge. The provider's knowledge is partially dependent upon where the diplomas were earned in years past, but more importantly by just how much time he or she has spent in study over the previous three months. Can a corporation, a hospital, an insurance company or a pharmaceutical company have a knowledge base? Only insofar as these legal entities promote and protect the agency of their individual providers and scientists.

The next element in building trust, is the willingness to act with integrity and to speak the truth. I am always amazed at what unpleasant truths and sensitive areas, I can touch on without offense being taken. Issues of obesity and overweight are touchy areas, but that conversation is usually welcomed by the patient. Men are supposed to be stoic, and to have control over their private emotions. Sometimes men have an angry demeanor, so that is where I go. I am always surprised when I ask a "macho" man who is angry, if he fights back tears frequently. Commonly he takes pause to consider, and he may soon be in tears in my office. Patients may want or expect antibiotics, but they more want to hear why that may not be the best solution. The patient may not want surgery, but sometimes that is the best solution, and they want to know why. Speaking the truth to patients works greatly to obtain their respect and their trust. The best interests of the patient should always be the first consideration. Transparency in cost is a step implied by this consideration. If the medication has side effects, discuss them. If the procedure is risky, make those risks known. That is physicianship.

A lot is said about always telling the truth. This is true most all the time, but sometimes delicacy is required. Longevity, prognosis, and mental competence can be point- blank topics. Generally, the patients will ask these questions when they are ready for the answers. The truth ought not to be a bludgeon. Saying nothing but the truth is different than a smack-down with the whole truth. If important management issues are at stake, hopefully family, friends, or social workers can be more fully informed.

On the other hand, in situations of advanced cancer or end-stage congestive heart failure conversations about the outlook are commonly wanted by the patient. At the end of our lives, we may welcome the end. I have had elderly patients, who at every visit expressed a wish to die, and in the ICUs, in their last minutes, we have celebrated that they are getting their desire.

The CAHPS data finds that patients appreciate facts, and solid explanations of the path suggested more than simply ordering what they expect or think they want. Compromises can be reached, but acquiescence to patient demands reduces that patient to a patron with a menu and the physician to a waiter. Some of my long-term patients requested hydroxychloroquine and ivermectin during our Covid-19 epidemic. No one got it from me. Caving to those demands would be a danger to the patient and an insult to the science upon which our field is based.

Another link in creating trust is communication, which entails a lot of listening and a little speaking. Being open to exploring emotional comments can be especially helpful in managing the care. Sometimes the diagnosis or management lies in the answer to a few specific questions and a directed physical exam. Limiting the time with the patient to asking those few questions or performing that limited examination can be quite time efficient for the provider but can thwart the patient's need to feel understood. Patience with a little rambling is advisable. It shows respect. If that rambling becomes truly excessive, which it can, finding a way to redirect without being offensive is a skill that must be developed by the practitioner. This comes with experience and gray hair.

The Relias Company and other healthcare advisory groups tout the routine use of the question, "What matters to you?" This basic question can lead to surprising answers, engendering truly patient centered management. Occasionally I have discounted the possibility of surgery in 90-plus year olds, only to find them more than ready to have the surgery to escape their pain. Sometimes patients want to leave the hospital prior to their doctors' plans. Issues of safety must be communicated with them, but ultimately the patient is in charge. Wading down into those weeds with the patient can prevent future misunderstandings and lawsuits. Asking "what matters to you" reestablishes who is setting the agenda.

Respect of the patient is another facet of trust that ought to be present. Quoting William Osler, "It is much more important to know what sort of a patient has a disease than what sort of a disease a patient has." Knowing who referred the patient, their family circle, their occupation, and where they live are all parts of common human interaction, and shows respect for the patient's individuality. Often patients are not distressed and may be unaware of any problems. During those visits, respect can be increased by pursuing broader knowledge of the patient. When the patient encounters a health problem, when referrals, medications, procedures, or hospitalizations are needed, the importance of a trusting relationship is maximal.

In visiting a physician, a background element of compassion is expected. For any number of reasons, sometimes valid, the provider may not like the patient. There is still a professional obligation to understand the problem from the patient's view, and to understand the humanity of that view. Drs. Stephen Trzeciak and Anthony Mazzarelli both practice at Cooper Medical School in New Jersey. They wrote a book, *Compassionomics*, published 2019. Their findings are quite extensively supported by the literature they reference, citing over 400 articles. This book details the many benefits of compassion, including improving the psychological and physical health of the patient, and the benefit to providers in decreasing burnout. A summary statement from a survey of 7 million online patient reviews says it well. "Healthcare consumers view healthcare first and foremost as a personal interaction." [7] and not just a medical transaction. The rat race of the medical-industrial complex does not promote personal interaction as an end goal.

A sixth characteristic of the trusted physician is that she or he is there for the long haul. This can be difficult in our mobile society, especially with spousal preferences sometimes changing plans, but within a few years after residency or fellowship, the physician and his family ought to be comfortable with the locale. Other people involved in healthcare, nurses, social workers, and administrators, as well as the patients, need to know the providers in the community they can count on... Many of my patients come to me complaining that they have been happy with the care they receive at a residents' clinic, but they tire of needing to get to know a new doctor every year. I have practiced in central Phoenix, Arizona, for 44 years now. I have been astounded by a local group of cardiologists who thought it was not important to have a known regular physician present at the office on a permanent basis. They rotate physicians through a variety of locations as needed to maximize the opportunities for procedures and the attendant reimbursement. The patients have not become aligned with that practice and I get an earful about this issue when they visit my office.

A final link in the trusted physician is that he or she runs, or is part of, a well-oiled machine. The support staff is happy, well-paid, stable, and committed to great patient care. If you are part of a large corporate practice, when problems occur, blaming the administration is convenient. It may be a valid reason, but it is not a valid excuse. Address those reasons.

All MBAs know the biggest part of a budget is personnel, so replacing people with technology will improve the bottom line. Right? Their first move is to develop phone trees. If you are looking for extra credit from your patients, have a person answer the phone. Recall the relief you feel when you call any office and a person answers the phone. If a person cannot answer the phone, be sure to call your office yourself on occasion to see if that phone tree is brief or insufferable.

In a well-run office the bills are paid, the facility is reasonably clean and comfortable, and perhaps interesting.

You start on time with functional systems. When a referral is made, your reputation is now dependent upon the workings of an outside system, which may not be very efficient. I work around that problem by texting that next doctor directly with the name, and number of the patient so he can work on the problem from inside her or his bureaucracy. And I ask that patient to call me in a week if an appointment has not been arranged. Using this texting system I just moved a patient's neurology appointment from two months away, to three days. As a safety net, I ask the patient to followup with me in ten days if an appointment has not been arranged.

None of these functionality issues are at the top of the patient experience list but they constitute a solid second place. Quite commonly patients will come to see me, saying the previous doctor was great but his office staff was incompetent. They could not trust that when a problem occurred, the office would not handle their needs and deliver a solution.

Corporate think is that bigger is better, because with the use of specialization, and of technology, efficiencies of size occur. This is true only to an extent. While those efficiencies increase arithmetically with the addition of specialized personnel, the attendant confusion increases exponentially throughout the organization. Moreover, oftentimes, the nursing and administrative staff will have more seniority than the physicians who may come and go in large organizations. The support staff may well be more interested in leaving at 5 p.m., than caring for the patients. The real benefit of mergers and increased size, in terms of power and income, accrues to those higher in the administrative food chain, the medical directors and the CEOs. So of course, these leaders will argue for growth. The question will that growth increase the trust in the physician. Usually not. Smaller, not bigger, is better. Smaller is more competent.

Corporate think is that advertisements and public relations, and buildings are to be embellished. As previous outlined, the core of patient experience is the relationship between the patient and the individual physician, not the external trappings.

In my opinion the primary way to optimal patient experience is to increase the trust in the provider. The seven features of the trusted physician are:

1) A solid knowledge base.

2) A commitment to acting with integrity and speaking the truth.

3) Open communication with the patient.

4) A genuine respect for the patient.

5) Acting with compassion.

6) Presence for the long haul.

7) Having a competently functioning office.

Trust is the key to the best patient experience.

Chapter 7

Population Health

Now it is the end of February 2022. On February 24th, the Russian army invaded Ukraine. This event was appalling to the Western world. We are riveted to news of battles in Ukraine and inspired by the bravery of the Ukrainian people. And we are reawakened to the preciousness of our liberty, and our opportunity to make a difference.

In this book, I have attempted to show the disadvantages of the for-profit corporate practice of medicine and the advantages of making maximal use of the talents of our physicians. We have discussed three of the quadruple aims: financial health, physician burnout, and patient experience. In this chapter I address the fourth aim: population health. One thread you will find in this chapter is the success local solutions have while national solutions falter.

There are a number of issues that determine the health of our population. Only one of them is having access to clinical medicine (medical personnel, hospitals, medications etc.) Problems of homelessness, hunger, violence, availability of nutritious food, and social determinants of health all contribute to poor health in our communities. We will delve into the struggles to create solutions, but first we need to grasp the scope of the problem.

HOMELESSNESS: In 2020 roughly 585,000 people were homeless in the United States, which works out to around 16 homeless per 10,000 people. This is per the United States Interagency Council on Homelessness. The USICH consists of representatives of 19 federal agencies, (including the Departments of Health and Human Services, Education, Veteran's Affairs, Justice, Homeland Security and others.) Per their homepage, "It works with federal, state, and local governments as well as the private sector to help communities create partnerships, use resources in the most efficient way, and employ evidence-based best practices." As we shall see, public health solutions to homelessness are determined more at the local or state level than at the Federal level.

Of these 585,000 homeless in the U.S., 27.9% live in California, a rate of 41 homeless people per 10,000 residents. My state, Arizona, has 15 homeless per 10,000; Texas 9 per 10,000; Mississippi 4 per 10,000; Alabama 6 per 10,000; and

New York State 45 per 10,000 population.

There are certainly medical consequences or associations of homelessness such as cardiopulmonary disease, skin diseases, sleep deprivation, mental illness, physical and sexual assault, drug dependency, etc. Also there is personal and psychological damage, such as loss of self-esteem, loss of ability and will to care for oneself, and increased risk of entering the criminal justice system. Once homelessness commences, there is shame and a loss of will to deal with the situation. This gives rise to a need to act quickly for those newly homeless, before hopelessness sets in.

HUNGER: Most of the following comes from the website of Feeding America. One in eight Americans (42 million) face food insecurity annually. This includes one in six children. Between 2008 and 2019 there was a roughly 7% drop in childhood food insecurity in the United States, from 22% to 18%. Because of unemployment with the Covid pandemic, childhood hunger went back up 5%. The consequences of food insecurity are both physical and mental. We see more diabetes, hypertension, and obesity. Hungry children are apt to have difficulty with schoolwork and with behavioral issues.

Feeding America is the largest hunger relief organization, and the second largest charitable organization in the U.S. It is a nonprofit company consisting of a network of over 200 food banks across America. Its history is instructive. In the late 1960s a retired businessman, John Van Hengel, was a volunteer in a soup kitchen here in Phoenix. He met a mother rummaging through garbage bins behind grocery stores to feed her children. She suggested there could be food banks where leftover produce could be stored and distributed. Mr. Van Hengel established St. Mary's food bank in 1967. My wife and I have contributed monthly for over 20 years. From the beginning it was successful and other communities noticed. By 1977 there were food banks in 18 cities across the nation. Van Hengel created a national organization of these food banks, America's Second Harvest. In 2008 this network changed its name to Feeding America. In 2020 Feeding America's goal is to create a hunger free America. It has a special intention of reaching out to traditionally indigent groups, and to rural communities, to addressing the root causes of poverty, and to supporting global efforts to address hunger.

Note Feeding America was not born in Washington, D.C. It grew from a great idea from a dumpster diver and a businessman, in the conservative state of Arizona.

HEALTH INSURANCE: Another factor contributing to population health issues in the U.S. is that many people have no health insurance at all. According to the Centers for Disease Control and Prevention, in the first six months of 2021, 31.1 million people in America, 9.6% of the population, did not have insurance for regular healthcare. For people under 65 years old, before Medicare applies, the figure is 11%. [3] When people without health insurance get ill or are injured, they are not ignored in our society. They are taken to emergency rooms and perhaps hospitalized. Then they are discharged, usually without continuity of care or ongoing measures of preventative care. This is an expensive effort, but enough money is built into the system that the hospitals do not go out of business. The taxpayers in America and the insurance customers, that is you and I, finance this shortfall. It would be better, much less expensive, and more world-class, if preventive care and ongoing follow-up were available to everyone.

Recently I spoke with two young women, Sonora Crittenden and Desiree De Melo, who work with the Community Benefit and Health Equity Department of our local St. Joseph's Hospital. They are experts in the delivery of public health support at the ground level. This department must submit a report every three years to the federal government about what the greatest community needs are and outline plans to help with these needs. They work with many local organizations to create these plans. One of their philosophies is to utilize "navigators" or clinical coordinators, who are familiar with or from the population they serve. By utilizing culturally, racially and linguistically similar workers, suspicions of the efforts of formal organizations are decreased.

So far, I have covered three major areas of social determinates of health, homelessness, food insecurity, and formal healthcare. Other major areas, where people commonly falter have to do with transportation, paying utilities, exposure to violence and having adequate education. Most people with one problem have multiple problems. Ms. Crittenden and Ms. De Melo, also point out that there are hundreds of local not-for-profit organizations dedicated to filling these various concerns. One of their biggest needs is for increased coordination of care. Our local Health Information Exchange, whose primary purpose is to connect doctors' offices with hospitals for the ready exchange of information, including hospital discharge summaries, is beginning a program where people in need of social services can be registered, be referred to the appropriate agency, and their outcomes tracked. These women with the Community Benefits Department also point out a surprising statistic. Forty percent of a person's health is determined by socio-economic factors; 30% by health behaviors; 20% by the healthcare they receive; and 10% is determined by their physical environment.

There is a lot of need for population health in the U.S. And, there is a lot of local talent, in non-profit organizations acting with agency, trying to better the big picture of healthcare in America. If Bernie Sanders' vision of national healthcare for all cannot be attained, perhaps the effort belongs under the radar, at the local level of the non-profit organizations. Perhaps some of that young enthusiasm and vision of medical students and young doctors and even older doctors, can be of benefit to this local effort.

Let's take a more formal look at Public Health in the United States. A recent series in the New England Journal regarding Public Health in America, published in late 2021, through early 2022 gives an excellent overview. It consists of eight brief articles covering the importance, the legalities and politics, and the epidemiologic science of population health. As it turns out, I needed to learn a lot. Honestly it has been a humbling experience, and an eye-opener. For instance, did you know that between 1900 and 2000, the life expectancy of the American male increased by 30 years? Medical science and the efforts of doctors and nurses and hospitals account for five of those years. Twenty-five of these years are due to the improvements in the public health arena. These improvements include improved sewage and other sanitation systems, clean water, rural electrification, improved communications, and better housing. [(3)] In 2018, we in America spent $93 billion on Public Health and $3.6 trillion on direct medical services. So, during the last century 83% (25/30) of our improvement in life span was instigated by the 2.5% (93 B/3.6 T) of the money allotted to public health measures. Ninety-seven and half percent of the money is in clinical medicine, the part attractive to the for-profit corporations dealing in healthcare, and it accounts for only 17% of the improvement.

A particularly helpful article in this series was written by David Hunter. [(5)] This paper includes a Venn Diagram showing the relationships of public health, our healthcare system, and our clinical efforts. Public health effects many measures including our clean water supply, sanitation, our responses to natural disasters, and infectious disease control; and it completely encompasses our healthcare system. The healthcare system includes the training of healthcare professionals, the availability of hospitals and medications, and the availability of public health organizations. The healthcare system completely encircles clinical medicine which has to do with the treatment of disease throughout the life course. What we doctors do, which is clinical medicine, which consumes so much of our attention and our finances, is just a small fraction of the big picture of our healthcare system.

One distinction, I never took time to consider is the difference between public health and population health. It goes something like this. Population health information is the science - the epidemiological science - upon which public health organizations act. People and groups can choose not to follow the advice because we presume to live in a liberated nation. But not following educated sound advice usually is not a great way to play your cards.

Interesting questions arise out of this dilemma. During our current Covid pandemic "anti-vaxxers" refuse Covid vaccines, for a variety of reasons, and it does seem to me that individuals can properly expect to not be assaulted with a needle against their will. On the other hand, hundreds of thousands of people have needlessly died of Covid infections, because refusing this vaccination directly contributed to the deaths, and to the lack of herd immunity. It also seems reasonable to me, that an individual can properly expect that he and his loved ones will be protected from an avoidable illness, when a safe and inexpensive method of protection is available. In our society this dilemma is left to our governmental systems and legal minds to adjudicate. More on this later.

This dilemma does not stop with Covid vaccinations. Dr. Tom Frieden was the director of the CDC between 2009 and 2017. He founded and is now the CEO of Resolve to Save Lives, an organization which aims to decrease cardiovascular death and to decrease epidemics in our world. He published an article on, March, 26 2022, in the Review Section of the Wall Street Journal [(6)], detailing how public health measures could decrease cardiovascular death. This is a short but superb article and is well worth our attention. He focuses on the role smoking, hypertension, and air pollution play in causing cardiovascular disease. To closely paraphrase, in the first two years of the Covid pandemic, it killed 900,000 people in the U.S. During those years atherosclerotic events, strokes and myocardial infarctions, killed 1.6 million. Three of the primary causes of these events are tobacco use, excessive salt intake, and air pollution. (He does not go into the role elevated cholesterol plays, as that is not especially amenable to public health measures.)

There are legislative steps society could take to decrease these factors, without any effort or sense of loss on the part of individuals. Nicotine addiction is a prime example. I have spent my career imploring patients to stop smoking. They nod yes, then light up on their way to their car in the parking lot. Later, I try to help them while watching them die of cancer, emphysema, or heart attacks. But public health measures work, whereas clinical medicine fails. It is well demonstrated that increasing the taxes on smoking drastically decreases smoking rates. It has been shown that when taxes are raised on cigarettes, the incidence of smoking decreases. If the tax is high enough, say $20 a pack, very few people smoke, and even fewer get started. Where clinical efforts fail, public health measures succeed. Why do we not tax cigarettes at a rate that demonstratively decreases smoking behavior? Why do we not tax cigarettes at a rate commensurate with the financial and social damage they do to our society? You know why. Because the tobacco industry throws up strong legal and political challenges. *

Hypertension is highly correlated with sodium intake and is a

---

* When I was in eighth grade, 1963, all the kids in my school were given small packs of five cigarettes. Of course, I had to man up and despite a little coughing and vomiting, I succeeded in smoking that first cigarette. It became a valuable juvenile social skill and a pack a day habit as a sophomore in college. I stopped as a senior in medical school. What a great investment by big tobacco. Five cigarettes for a potentially life-long addict.

prime cause of atherosclerosis. I spend a lot of time treating hypertension and asking my patients to decrease their salt use. But salt at the table accounts for less than 10% of our daily salt intake. Individuals' actions will not solve the problem. Most salt intake comes from commercially prepared packaged foods. The food companies think, they need that salt ingredient to remain competitive. But a reduction of 30% of our salt intake would stop around 50,000 premature deaths in the U.S. annually, and consumers would hardly notice the decrease in their food. (Wow! 50,000 lives.) Front of package labeling of salt content gives consumers a chance to decrease salt intake on their own, and is prominent in some countries, (e.g., Chile, Mexico, and Israel.) The food industry clearly resists these changes in the U.S. Again, public health measures can work where individual efforts fail.

Dr. Frieden points out that a third cause of premature cardiovascular disease is air pollution. This was a surprising finding to me, as we don't hear much about this in clinical medicine. Particulate matter less than 2.5 microns (PM2.5) annually accounts for around 3,000,000 deaths globally. America is making progress in reducing PM2.5, in part from the Clean Air Act of the Nixon administration in the 1970s. Again, individual action cannot affect the air we inhale. But a great deal has been done and can be done with governmental action. We are actively decreasing our reliance on fossil fuels and moving to renewable energy, including home roof top solar systems and electric vehicles. In part this occurs, because of a push from public health agencies, resulting in governmental regulations.

In summarizing, Dr. Frieden writes, "Will the Covid pandemic usher in an era of opposition to all governmental public-health measures? Perhaps, but it might also lead to a recognition that some public-health actions are essential because, without them, there is no practical way for individuals to control their own health risks...we may come to see that the problem isn't government action but rather inaction in the face a deadly disease's obvious causes."

Whence the inaction?

For the last 20 years or so, the red/blue divide has become more fractious, obviously, and this is part of the problem. In that JAMA series mentioned at the start of this chapter, one of the articles reviews the historic legal foundations of U.S. public health law. This article was written by Michelle Mello, J.D, and Wendy Parmet, J.D., [(7)] both from Stanford University. Their reach goes back a long way, to rights established in our founding constitution, and its amendments.

"Historically, public health law has largely been state law. In 1824, in Gibbons v Ogden, the Supreme Court recognized that states had plenary power—or "police power" — that includes the power to enact "health laws of every description.

"State laws can be preempted, or overridden, by conflicting federal laws ... all laws must respect constitutionally protected individual rights, including free speech, free exercise of religion, procedural due process, equal protection (protection from discrimination), and some aspects of privacy."

This article then reviews the role our courts play in adjudicating real time conflicts, including vaccination rights, liberty from quarantine for infectious people, mental health, civil confinement, the right to bear arms, and the right to privacy including restrictions on abortion.

“Traditionally, courts have granted substantial deference to scientific experts, and government officials about measures needed to protect health. That deference appears to be waning, in numerous doctrinal areas.

“Though unsettling, these developments are unsurprising in light of our country’s increasing political polarization (which extends to judicial appointments) … A broad social reckoning is underway regarding how much power officials should have to restrict liberties in the name of public health.”

Dr. Steven Woolf, from University of Virginia, has brought this reckoning into focus with our Covid epidemic.

(8) As I pointed out in the beginning chapters, people living in America have a disadvantage in terms of life expectancy, compared to other advanced nations, and this disadvantage is increasing. The gap in 2010 was 1.9 years, and in 2020 it was 4.7 years. There also is a gap in longevity between the red and the blue states. This gap was true of all racial and ethnic groups. Citing 2022 information from the CDC, Dr. Woolf points out that middle age (25-64-year olds) mortality differed by a factor of 228% in non-Hispanic White individuals in states with the highest mortality rates (571 per 100,000) compared to the states with the lowest (250 per 100,000). This difference is explained in large part by a growing polarization in public policies between red and blue states. When cigarettes are taxed at a higher rate, smoking deaths decrease. When motorcycle helmet laws are relaxed, injury deaths increase.

When the Covid epidemic hit, the public health response differed greatly between more liberal, and more conservative states. States with larger amounts of vaccine resistance had much higher death rates compared to states with higher vaccination rates.

This was true with the Delta wave and again with the Omicron variant.

Dr. Woolf continues, "In contrast (to more liberal states), states that had spent decades opposing public health provisions were among the most resistant to Covid-19 guidelines and took active measures to resist restrictions. Some elected officials made a political issue out of challenging scientific evidence, embracing dubious theories, and labeling public health safeguards as infringement on personal freedom." [8]

In agreement with the attorneys from Stanford, Mello and Parmet, Dr. Woolf points out that state control of the health and safety of their citizens is increasing. "The implications of these state-level actions require medical and public health professionals, and the public shift their focus from the political standoffs in Washington, D.C., to the escalating activity in state capitols and to be vigilant about policies that threaten health and safety, deepen inequities, or target vulnerable groups."

Right. Another revelation. Honestly, I have given up on the notion that our elected leaders in Washington D.C. can find any functional common ground. Let them posture, pontificate, and argue while the locals solve the problems.

Last night I reviewed the latest JAMA issue, May, 05th 2022. In it there is a Viewpoint by Dr. Don Berwick, [9] "Getting Serious about Producing Health the Ten Teams Challenge." This is the same Don Berwick that produced the Triple Aim concept in 2008 at the Institute for Healthcare Improvement. He is now a Senior Fellow with the Institute, which is based in Boston. In this statement he reviews many of the points made in this chapter. The healthcare industry accounts for only 10% of the variation in health found in America. He points out that 50% of the variation is determined by genetics and 40% is dictated by social determinants of health. Our healthcare industry will soon spend 20% of our national GNP (far more than other first world nations and gives us inferior results.) The focus of these ten teams would be addressing: health coverage, food security, housing security, immigrant needs, corrections, and prison health, climate and de-carbonization, voting rights, education support, early childhood support, and elderly, and loneliness issues. "Absent a forcing function from government, that (significant funding) can and should begin with voluntary changes in the priorities and strategies of hospitals and other healthcare organizations… The Ten Teams idea is not for healthcare to take control, but rather to be a generous and active participant in community-led activities to improve social determinants."

This is where I wind up this chapter on population health. It is important, more important than clinical healthcare, to our nation's well-being. There is not a fortune to be made in solving population health issues, so the for-profit corporations will not belong here. Our leadership in Washington D.C., cannot provide a way forward. There is a great deal of local activity and agency aiming to address our healthcare problems. These efforts could benefit from the involvement of healthcare providers. And healthcare providers can find meaning and fulfillment in supporting these efforts.

We physicians do not have to be consumed by our existence on the medical-industrial treadmill.

Chapter 8
Going Forward

Today is January 1st, 2023, and something seems to be in the air. This winter's holiday season seemed a little more hopeful than those of the last three years. We have settled in with the Covid pandemic as it becomes less virulent, if more contagious. The midterm elections are over and some words of reconciliation between the right and the left are making the news. The brave citizens of Iran continue their marches, looking for their freedom. Against all odds the citizens of Ukraine fight to maintain their independence and freedom. Change is in the air.

American medicine will soon shift as its central and most influential player, Medicare, will need refinancing and rebuilding in 2024. We need to take this period as an opportunity to discuss our entire healthcare system. Why? This book has addressed that question in some detail. Again, taking the quadruple aim as the rubric, our healthcare is twice as expensive as the average of all first world countries. Patients are tired of being treated as profit centers, as diagnoses, instead of as individual people. Roughly 10% of our population have no health insurance coverage at all. And after all the effort and expense of becoming a physician, many find no fulfillment, and leave the profession for happier careers. My attorney patient mentioned in the introduction is right. Our healthcare system is on fire. There is much to improve.

What specifically needs to happen? We need to evolve into a single-payor healthcare system. We need a much higher percentage of primary care physicians. To the extent possible, the profit motive needs to be rooted out of healthcare. The human values of the people we admit into medical schools ought to be cultivated throughout their training and beyond. As our medical students progress through their training and enter the work force, they should be positioned to change, not join, the medical-industrial complex. The changes that I have listed here are apt to take years to achieve, but a great deal has been done already to point us in the right direction. It needs to be acknowledged that the whys and hows of improving healthcare in America is an ongoing evolving process. Every week, I scan the JAMA and other literature. Every week another article appears that could easily be incorporated into this book.

So how do we move ahead? Regarding our evolution into a single-payor system, resistance from the private insurance companies will be major, as it has been in the past. They would be happy with no change at all. And our healthcare systems are too complicated, and widely interwoven for an abrupt change to occur. Public option insurance as an alternative to private insurance would create some real competition in the healthcare market, and provide some time for evolution and growth. Seasoned management recruited from the private sector to establish policies and reimbursement levels would be necessary. Please note that Medicare reimbursement levels are widely accepted by hospitals and physicians, and these rates are much lower than rates of private insurance in commercial markets. The goal of the public option would be to provide less expensive healthcare insurance and gradually supplant private industry. It is critical that this option be a financial success. Given that constitutionally healthcare is governed at the state level, the public option likely will begin with state management. It already exists in three states, Nevada, Colorado, and Washington.

There is a widely recognized need for more primary care providers in the U.S. This need is frequently emphasized in Congress and in our medical journals. Our oversupply of specialists with all their procedures, drives up the entire cost of healthcare. The flood of chronic healthcare problems our nation-faces, hypertension, diabetes, congestive heart failure, depression, obesity, etc. - cannot be handled by specialists alone. There are not enough specialists for that long-term management, nor is their expertise broad enough. A great deal of health problems can be handled, indeed in a superior fashion, at the primary care level. However, our lack of primary care providers undermines public health efforts and the achievement of equity in medicine. Some argue that increasing the number of nurse practitioners would suffice. Certainly, nurse practitioners have excellent training and bring good judgement to their work. However, the training experience of hospital internships and residencies, lasting at least three years, places the MDs and DOs at a distinct advantage over the NPs in assessing, and managing the array of serious health problems that can walk through the door. In my mind, a partnership of physicians working side by side with NPs is optimal.

Why do our numbers of primary care physicians lag? As pointed out in the chapter on physician experience, the reimbursement in primary care medicine is far less than in the specialty world. The rate of reimbursement is largely established by the recommendations rendered by the Relative Value Scale Update Committee (RUC) of the American Medical Association. (1) CMS does not have to follow these recommendations, but usually does. This committee is comprised of many specialties in American Medicine and was established in 1992. The majority of the members are indeed specialists. Surgeons and other proceduralists are represented by 18 members: primary care medicine by four.

Note that the American Medical Association is a prominent name in the United States. It promotes itself as the voice of American Physicians. More accurately, it is the voice of American Specialists. CMS, with the backing of our Federal Government, pays a great deal of attention to the AMA. But less than twenty percent of practicing physicians in America belong to the AMA. [2]

Per their website, the AMA does say they are trying to promote primary care medicine. They have said so since the RUC's beginning in 1992. Evidently, given the ongoing and widespread acknowledgement that much more primary care medicine is needed, the AMA has failed in their promotion. The book by Miriam Laugensen, *Fixing Medical Prices: How Physicians Are Paid*, [3] details the problem with the RUC, in which the specialists protect their elevated reimbursement at the expense of primary care. Thirty-one years of failure is enough. It is time to discontinue the Revenue Update Committee. CMS works ultimately at the direction of the U.S. Federal Government. The Federal Government could direct that CMS completely disregard the RUC and develop its own methods of determining medical fees.

Really people, the emperor has no clothes. The AMA is an institution in the United States. It publishes JAMA, the most commonly cited journal in this book. Everyone knows how important the AMA is, but its RUC is the problem that is stopping competitive reimbursement of primary care medicine. It is the main reason we have a shortage of primary care doctors. And that is the primary reason we are not moving forward in achieving the quadruple aim. Going along with things because the AMA is so powerful and is so interwoven in our system is called complicity. Please let your legislators know your thoughts.

The stock market should not be involved in the practice of medicine. Our police departments and fire departments, which are utilities, are not expected to return a profit for shareholders. Arguably, healthcare is a similar utility. Everyone needs it on occasion, at times just as urgently as policemen or fire fighters are needed. Pressures to increase productivity or decrease necessary procedures by physicians should not be influenced by the return on investment for shareholders.

Reimbursement for most medical visits and procedures are already controlled, or pegged to the Medicare reimbursement schedule. Within that context, as transparency becomes more the norm, there should be little room for profit from purely financial investments. The delivery of healthcare at the granular level is a private and personal event. Large hospital systems, medical and pharmaceutical research, and the education of medical personnel all require organized and complex teamwork, and such organizations need to be financially supported, but not to the extent that the CEOs of our major medical insurance companies are given multimillion dollar annual compensations, and not to the extent that shareholders profit from these companies, while needed procedures and medications are denied to patients.

The human values of the entering medical students are to be encouraged. The pressures of academia and the responsibilities of providing knowledgeable healthcare to patients is tremendous. This pressure tempers students and residents into serious people. During this process, these human values potentially can be replaced with the values of MBAs, and the focus on making money, so characteristic of the medical-industrial complex. It becomes the water most medical personnel swim in, so ubiquitous we do not even notice how greed affects our practices. There is no room for the fulfillment of providing a meaningful medical service. This is exactly the moral injury Dr. Wendy Dean is writing about as the root cause of medical burnout.

So, these are the goals I suggest we move toward. How we get there depends on the different roles people play in healthcare.

CMS: Arguably the most powerful people in healthcare, th biggest difference makers, work within CMS. This agency suggests the laws and regulations most hospitals and providers follow. It provides the models many of our insurances emulate. Ideas, discussions, writings abound throughout healthcare; CMS distills them and promulgates them into reality. Think pay for value and shared savings.

The biggest mistake from CMS is that primary care physicians are paid much less for their time than doctors in the specialties. As reviewed in the chapter on agency, the time spent in training and the malpractice risk is higher in the specialties. Some difference is appropriate. But not to the extent that anesthesiologists average an income of

$800,000 per year, more than three times higher than primary care doctors, and spend much less time doing it. One metric that could be used to determine reimbursement is the downstream dollars the practice influences. Another is the downstream responsibility. When the patient has recovered from his surgery, the surgeon is done. Not so for the PCP, where the responsibility lasts a lifetime. They should be paid for this responsibility. As previously stated, the Update Committee of the AMA has failed and needs to be disbanded.

Also, CMS ought to place the small private practices on an equal financial footing with the hospital employed doctors. The private practitioner should be paid as much as the hospital employed practitioner for the same service, not less.

There are efficiencies of size, and smaller practices should be permitted to band together for purchasing strength, contract negotiations, and easing flow of information, without forming formal corporations. This is already beginning in the accountable care organizations, and in state- wide Information Exchange Programs.

Another influence that CMS should adopt is to reward stability. The patient experience is severely damaged, when they are treated like widgets on a conveyer belt. Human beings enjoy working with personalities with whom they are familiar. Granted, shuffling physicians around to mine the procedural opportunity of the day may make sense to MBAs, but patients and physicians don't like it. Once a physician establishes a location, a small percentage of reimbursement could be used to keep him there. A physician ought to be or become an institution in him or herself, of acknowledged value to the community. We will not get there if we permit the medical-industrial complex, with its emphasis on milking more and more money out of the system, to overwhelm the intrinsic morality of physicians.

In trying to promote physician experience, and decrease burnout, CMS should standardize the metrics that the big insurance companies expect the physician practices to achieve. The data set expected of physicians, used to reward insurance companies for annual physical exams, needs to be the same for CIGNA, Humana, Aetna, UHC, etc. As I pointed out in chapter 2, Silos, the decision tree of physicians is complex enough without needing to worry about what insurance the patient has.

Finally, Medicare should promote an insurance option for everyone – all ages. There is no need to outlaw the big five national companies. Let them wither. Just create a little real competition and support its growth. This begins by pushing forward the "public option," run by the states, in which the for-profit insurance companies would finally get some actual competition.

The wants of our population are seemingly endless. Patients may say they want surgery scheduled when they please, they want only brand name drugs, and to have their babies delivered by C-Section, when they find it most convenient, and lumbar spine MRIs when a plain film would suffice. But caving to these demands would destroy the financial competitive edge a public program ought to have. A public option insurance company would have some intrinsic financial advantages, including spending less on advertising, less on influencing our politicians, and less on administration. The public option oversight boards could be comprised of people interested in saving money, ensuring transparency, and staying in the black. It could have access

to large physician networks as participation in other public programs, such as Medicare and Medicaid, could be contingent on participation in the public option insurance companies.

GOVERNMENT: Our governmental representatives, at both the state and national level, stamp the laws we all must follow. They take the suggestions of CMS, other experts, and of vested interests, and craft them into law. They have a moral obligation to ensure that fair laws are promoted. Just as they ensure that primary providers are not gifted for prescriptions written, and there is no kickback for referrals, they have an obligation to be sure they themselves receive no undue gifts, kickbacks, or campaign contributions for votes - that constitutes bribery. Taking campaign contributions from for-profit medical insurance companies, or consortiums of such companies is immoral.

Health insurance corporations should not have the freedom to change their offerings every year, as this can be confusing to the patients and disruptive to patient physician relationships. As an interim step, until a single-payor system evolves, healthcare insurance companies should be restricted to three- or four-year contracts with the doctors, the hospital systems, and the patients. These regulations fall to our elected representatives.

Finally, the goals of the quadruple aim are interwoven and all four goals simultaneously should be at the forefront of creating governmental medical regulations. Laws affecting any one of the aims will affect the other three as well.

MEDICAL STUDENTS AND RESIDENTS: Medical students are the most important part of the solution. Please understand that you are not an imposter. You are the future leaders of healthcare, and you will have something to contribute. Your family is immensely proud of you. In part they are proud because you are an opportunity to carry their most important family values into the future. That you are in your position demonstrates your intellectual prowess, and humanitarian strength. Certainly, medical school will challenge your intellect. Let your many experiences in medical school embellish your altruism.

As you progress through your years, especially in rotations with private doctors, keep your eyes open. See how different systems care for the different patients. Beware of easy paths as they always come with a price. You are studying to become part of a noble, esteemed, and responsible profession. American healthcare needs you to be active in shaping its future. Do not be a pawn. Bear the complexity of the quadruple aim in mind, when making your decisions.

Residents are going through the toughest part of medical training. This exposure to the weight of responsibility, this tempering, separates you from paramedical personnel. During residency there is little time to think about larger social issues. However, bear in mind that it is absolutely possible to have a successful career without caving to the for-profit corporate practice of medicine. You lose a lot when signing up with large corporate providers of healthcare.

MEDICAL EDUCATORS: No disrespect here, but remember the bigger context, and what you are doing. You are molding the future leadership of medicine in the United States. As has been made quite clear, there are major problems in medical care in the United States. Take a step back, and recognize that your underlying mission is to improve healthcare in the United States. Become an expert in the issues of the quadruple aim and explore these issues with your students. Most students are not going to become researchers or subspecialists in your field of medicine. Most will go into non-academic practice and will shape, with their career decisions, the future of healthcare. Discussing the goals for our society's healthcare system, and considering solutions, should be an ongoing major component of the curriculum of medical students.

PRACTICING PHYSIANS: Yes, medicine is a demanding taskmaster. That is what you signed up for and you worked very hard to get here. Now, those demands may be overwhelming. If you are depressed, please seek psychiatric help. I personally have been on antidepressants for more than 20 years. If you are disillusioned, consider a change. The for-profit corporations do not own you, and they should not be the source of moral injury. You fill a valued and responsible role in society, and you deserve to find fulfillment in your work.

There are literally hundreds of not-for-profit organizations that could use your support and expertise. The challenge of the Ten Teams approach may provide a gratifying use of your abilities. I personally do not think more time off for meditation or counselling is the answer to burnout. Dr. Stephen Covey, author of *The 7 Habits of Highly Effective People*, (3) has written about the distinction of distress and eustress ("good stress."). The challenge is not to escape responsibilities but to engage them in a fulfilling way. Seek a problem that you can embrace and fully use your energy, knowledge, and talents.

I am a solo practitioner of general internal medicine, and find it fulfilling. I no longer visit patients in the hospitals, largely because of the time demands of maintaining electronic medical records in my office. I have worked in Central Phoenix for over forty years now. Most of the time, I take my own call. Once or twice a year, when traveling, I trade call with another generalist. My office works four days a week. We accept Medicare insurance rates and multiple insurances. A variety of patients are seen, from the indigent to jet setters. And we see our patients same day or next, depending on the circumstances. There are four full-time employees, all of whom have been with the practice for over two years. I am not a great businessman, but with help from my wife and my staff, I stay in business. My employees help me with the computers. I have time for social and volunteer activities, and exercise. It is possible to make all this work.

HEALTHCARE CORPORATIONS: The large healthcare

insurance companies, especially the for-profit ones, manage a great deal of wealth. A quick stroll through Siri is instructive regarding the salaries of the top CEOs in healthcare: Humana

$16.4 M, Anthem $17.1 M, United Healthcare $18.9 M, CIGNA $19.7 M, and AETNA $27.9 M. These are all for- profit healthcare companies. Note the vice-presidents of these corporations commonly make more than a million dollars per year.

I do not wish these leaders ill, personally, but I do think they have lost their way. When the United States leads the world in healthcare expense, and lags the entire first world in quality of healthcare; when healthcare expense is the largest cause of bankruptcy in the U.S.; when 9.6% of our population has no formal healthcare at all; a major restructuring is due. The Milton Friedman ethos of profit being the sole purpose of a corporation, is backwater. I do not know if this means Medicare for All is the answer, but it seems to be the most likely candidate. Other structures are possible, and may evolve from the local ground up, rather than from Washington, D.C. down. If a public option insurance plan were to appear, whose primary intent was not profitability, it could take root, and outgrow the current for- profit plans.

MASS MEDIA: The news outlets have a role to play here. As we have seen the Right/Left divide is a major problem. The juicy polemics may help sell your newspapers or television programs; however you have a higher calling than sensationalism. I believe there is a need to avoid the put-downs, the oversimplifications, and to promote both sides of the story. Your first obligation is to provide the unvarnished facts. The Right and Left will never meet unless both start from a common ground of facts. As I have pointed out, both the Right and the

Left encourage saving money. Both sides can see that reliance on emergency rooms for basic healthcare needs is a waste of money.

GENERAL POPULATION: You are, of course, what this is all about. Sooner or later, everybody will need healthcare. Many of the solutions to our healthcare issues have to do with correcting the social determinants of health. There are many organizations dedicated to solving these problems. Just as you have a civic responsibility to vote, and to generally perform acts of kindness, you have an obligation to support local efforts to help the unfortunate. The for- profit corporations have no business in healthcare. As we have seen, a single-payor system would be of benefit. Be sure your governmental representatives know how you feel.

The need for change in healthcare is evident. With the financial difficulties facing Medicare, now is a particularly good time to reexamine our entire system. There are steps we can take.

We can move forward and achieve the quadruple aim.

Footnotes

Chapter 1. Introduction

1. *Being Wrong – Adventures in the Margin of Error*
Kathryn Schulz, 2010

2. "The Triple Aim: Care, Health, and Cost"
Donald Berwick, Thomas Nolan, John Whittington
Health Affairs, Vol. 27, No. 3, 2008

3. "From Triple to Quadruple Aim: Care of the Patient Requires Care of the Provider"
Thomas Bodenheimer, Christine Sinsky
Annals of Family Medicine, Vol. 12, No. 6, 2014.

4. "The State of the U.S. Health System in 2022 and the Outlook for 2023."
Dingel, Hanna, et. al. 12-22-22
Peterson-KFF Health Systems Tracker: Access and Affordability

Chapter 2. Silos

1. *Deadly Spin*
   Wendell Potter, 2010

2. "The 10 Highest Paid CEOs at Publicly Traded Health Insurance Companies"
   Andrew Cass
   Beckers Healthcare, Payer Issues, August 2022

3. "Centers for Medicare and Medicaid Services Salaries 2021"
   Federal Pay.org.

4. "U.S. Public Health Law—Foundation and Emerging Shifts"
   Michelle Mello, Wendy Parmet
   New England Journal of Medicine
   2022 Vol. 386: pp 805-808.

5. "Medicare and Medicaid: The Past as Prologue"
   Edward Berkowitz
   Healthcare Finance Review, 2005
   Vol. 27 No. 2: pp 11-23.

6. Peterson-KFF Health Systems Tracker.
   Health Spending Scoreboard
   11-26-2022

7. "Mirror, Mirror 2021, Reflecting Poorly"
The Commonwealth Fund: Improving Healthcare Quality, 8-4-21

8. World Health Organization Website
"Health Topics" 6-21-2000

9. "Beyond Burnout: The Real Problem Facing Doctors is Moral Injury"
Simon Talbot, Wendy Dean
- *Medical Economics*, 3-15-19

10. *Crossing the Quality Chasm: A New Health System for the 21ST Century*
The National Institute of Medicine 2001

11. "Accelerating Global Improvements in Healthcare Quality"
Leatherman and Berwick
JAMA 2020 Vol. 324, No. (24) pp 2479-2480

12. "Patient Consumerism, Healing Relationships, and Rebuilding Trust in Healthcare."
Khullar and Darlene
JAMA 2020 Vol. 324, No. (23) pp 2359-2360

13.” Reducing Administrative Waste in the U.S. Healthcare System”

R. Kocher
JAMA 2-2-2021 Vol. 325, No. (5) pp 427-428

14. “Surprise Billing: A Flashpoint for Major Policy Issues in Healthcare”

C. Colla JAMA 2-23-21 Vol. 325. No. (8) pp 715-716

Chapter 3. Agency

1. Med Edits 2022 Facts: Applicants and Matriculants Data

2. *Drive: The Surprising Truth About What Motivates Us,* Daniel Pink 2009

3. "Trends in Compensation of Primary Care Physicians Versus Specialist Physicians After Implementation of the Affordable Care Act" Hsiang, W. JAMA 7-28-2020, Vol. 3, No. (7)

4. *Fixing Medical Prices: How Physicians Are Paid,* Meriam Laugesen 2016

Chapter 4. Financial Health

1. "How Does Health Spending in the U.S. Compare to Other Countries?"

   Peterson-KFF Health Systems Tracker: Health Spending Scoreboard

   11-26-22

2. "Mirror, Mirror 2021, Reflecting Poorly"

   The Commonwealth Fund: Improving Healthcare Quality

   8-4-21

3. "Historical National Health Expenditure 2021"

   National Health Expenditure Data

   NHE Fact Sheet 2-17-23

4. *The Price We Pay,*

   Marty Makary 2019

5. "Factors Associated with Increases in U.S. Healthcare Spending."

   J. Dieleman
   JAMA 2017 Vol. 318, pp 1668-1678

6. "Is Single-Payor the Answer for the U.S. Healthcare System?"

   V. Fuchs
   JAMA 2018; Vol. 319, No. (1): 15-16

Chapter 5. Physician Well-being

1. "Taking Action Against Clinician Burnout: A Systems Approach to Professional Wellbeing"

    The National Academies of Science, Engineering, and Medicine, 2019

2. "Physician Suicide: A Call to Action"

    M. Kalmoe, et. al.

    Missouri Medicine Vol. 116, No. (3) May-June 2019

3. "I Cry But No One Cares": Physician Burnout and Depression Report 2023.

    L. Kane MA *Medscape Internal Medicine* 1- 20-2023.

4. "The Business Case for Investing in Physician Wellbeing"

    T. Shanafelt, C.Sinsky, et. al. *JAMA* 2017 Vol. 177, No. (12) pp 1826-1832.

5. "Cultural and Structural Features of Zero-Burnout Primary Care Practices"

    E. Samuels, et al.

    Health Affairs, June 2021, pp 928-936

6. "Rediscovering Meaning and Purpose: An Approach to Burnout in the Time of Covid-19 and Beyond"

    S. Southwick, et al. *The American Journal of Medicine* 5-11-21

7. *Man's Search for Meaning,*
Victor E. Frankl 1959 (page 99.)

8. *Drive: The Surprising Truth About What Motivates Us,*
D. Pink 2009

9. "Autonomy, Mastery, Respect, and Fulfillment are Key to Avoiding Moral Injury in Physicians"
S. Talbot and W. Dean Access the bmj.com, Jan. 16, 2020

Chapter 06. Patient Experience

1. "What is Patient Experience?"
Website, Agency for Healthcare Research and Quality. 2023.

2. "What Consumers Say About Their Experiences with their Health Plans and Medical Care"
CAHPS Health Plan Survey Data Base, 2019

3. "Should Healthcare Providers be Accountable for Patients' Care Experiences?"
R. Anhang Price, et. al.
Journal of General Internal Medicine, 2015, Feb. 30, No. (27) pp 253-256

4. "Patient Experience: Fundamentals and New Frontiers"
Relias, WhitePaper: *Improving Patient Care,* 2020

5. "Building Trust in Healthcare -- Why, Where, and How"
D. Khullar
JAMA 2019; Vol. 322, No. (6) pp 507-509

6. "Consumer Perspectives on Patient Experience"
J. Wolf, President, The Beryl Institute

7. *C ompassionomics*
S. Trzeciak, A. Massarelli
2019

Chapter 07. Population Health

1. "State of Homelessness"

   United States Interagency on Homelessness, Web site: 12-19-2022

2. "Our Vision: An America Without Hunger"

   Feeding America, Website: 2023

3. "Health Insurance Coverage"

   Center for Disease Control and Prevention

   National Center for Health Statistics 4-2023

4. Public Health In America

   New England Journal of Medicine: Series 2021 - 2022.

5. "The Complementarity of Public Health and Medicine -

   - Achieving the Highest Attainable Standard of Health"

   D. Hunter

   The New England Journal of Medicine Vol. 385; 6 pp 481-484.

6. "Stopping a Pandemic Deadlier Than Covid

   Tom Frieden

   The Wall Street Journal; Review March 26- 27, 2022

7. "U.S. Public Health Law -- Foundations and Emerging Shifts"

M. Mello and W. Parmet

The New England Journal of Medicine, Vol. 386; No. 9 pp 805-808

8. "The Growing Influence of State Governments on Population Health in the United States"

S. Woolf

JAMA 4-12-22 Vol. 327; No. 14, pp 1331-1332

9. "Ten Teams"

D. Berwick

JAMA Vol. 327; No. 19 pp 1865-1866

Chapter 08. Going Forward

1. *Fixing Medical Prices: How Physicians Are Paid*

   Meriam Laugesen 2016

2. "Is the AMA Really the Voice of Physicians in the U.S.?"

   L. Girgis *Physicians Weekly* 6-9-2015.

3. *The 7 Habits of Highly Effective People*

   Stephen Covey, 1989

Made in the USA
Monee, IL
04 November 2026

67374682R00069